To your health!

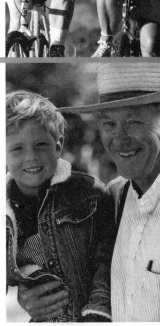

In an ongoing effort to promote better health and well-being, Merck-Medco Managed Care, L.L.C., is pleased to provide you with our new **Medication Guidebook for Older Adults**.

This handy reference booklet offers:

* Important information about a variety of common physiological and psychological conditions.

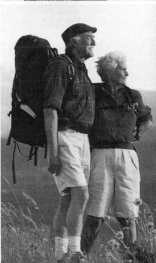

* The uses, effects, and side effects of the medications used to treat those conditions.

We hope you, as an older adult, find this guideline a valuable tool in maintaining your good health.

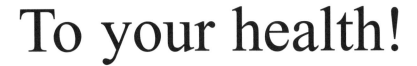

Partners For Healthy Aging™

EDITOR

Mark Monane, M.D., M.S., F.A.C.P., A.G.S.F.
Medical Policy & Programs
Merck-Medco Managed Care, L.L.C.

ASSOCIATE EDITORS
MERCK-MEDCO MANAGED CARE, L.L.C.

Gail A. Chirico
Department of Medical Affairs

Becky A. Nagle, Pharm.D., B.C.P.S.
Clinical Practice & Education
Clinical Practices & Therapeutics

Heather-Ann Periconi, R.Ph.
Utilization Management
Program Development

Ann M. Christiansen, Pharm.D.
Managed Care Resident

CONTRIBUTORS

Amita Dasmahapatra, M.D.
Medical Policy and Programs

Paul Greenberg, M.D.
Medical Policy and Programs

Alan Lotvin, M.D.
Medical Policy and Programs

George Fulop, M.D.
Medical Policy and Programs

Laurence J. Hirsch, M.D.
Medical Policy and Programs

Glen D. Stettin, M.D.
Utilization Management

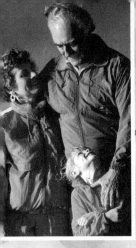

Contents

Introduction 2

Arthritis and Pain 10

Breathing Problems 30

Constipation 52

Depression 64

Diabetes. 82

Glaucoma 96

Heartburn, Indigestion, and Ulcers 112

Heart Disease and Chest Pain 136

Heart Failure 150

High Blood Pressure 160

Irregular Heartbeats 192

Irritable Bowel Syndrome 202

Osteoporosis 206

Parkinson's Disease 222

Sleep Problems and Nervousness 234

Stroke and Blood Clotting Prevention 250

Underactive Thyroid 262

Glossary 268

List of Brand Names and Manufacturers 270

Resources for Help and Information 280

Index 284

Personal Medication Record 294

Introduction

The use of modern medication has allowed people to live longer. Medications are very helpful for both treating and preventing many diseases in older people. However, older people may have some special needs when it comes to medication. In the sections to follow, we discuss why older people may have more side effects from medication, how growing older affects the way medication works for you, and some problems that can occur with prescription and over-the-counter (OTC) medications (those you can buy without a doctor's prescription). Also, we will discuss some common problems with taking medication that may come up for older people, information you need to know about your medications, and tips for taking medication in the safest way possible.

Side effects of medication in older people

Generally, the benefits of medications exceed their risks. However, sometimes medications can cause side effects, or unwanted problems. Common side effects from medications include constipation, dizziness, and headache. It may be hard to tell the difference between some side effects and the symptoms of certain diseases. For this reason a person may not know if he or she is having a side effect. For example, some medications may make it easier for people to fall or to become confused, side effects that some people might not know may be caused by the medications they are taking.

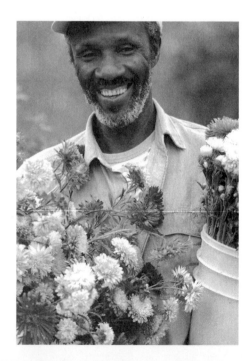

Side effects of medication occur more often in older people. There are many reasons why this is true. First, many older people have several diseases or conditions and,

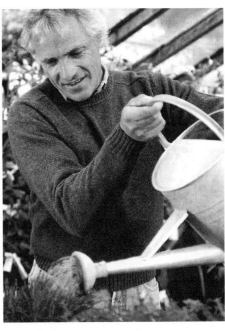

therefore, take several medications. The more medications a person is taking, the more likely he or she is to have side effects. Also, there is a greater chance that the medications will affect or interact with each other. Another important reason why older people have more side effects is that medications often act differently in the body as we age.

How growing older affects the way medication works

As a person grows older, many changes occur that are a normal part of aging. We know changes that occur on the outside of the body, such as wrinkles and gray hair. Changes also occur on the inside. Changes in the body organs, such as the kidneys and liver, can make a big difference in how medications are removed from the body.

First, it is important to know what happens when you take a medication. After the pill is swallowed, it goes into the stomach where the pill mixes with fluids and breaks down into small particles. Then the medication passes through the wall of the stomach or intestines and goes into the bloodstream. The blood carries the medication to a part of the body where it acts (for example, lowering blood pressure). Later, the medication is removed from the body. The kidney and liver are the two organs that remove medications from the body.

With aging, normal changes occur in the kidneys and the liver. Because of these changes, the kidneys and liver do not remove medications as well as they do in younger people. You can think of what happens to the body by comparing it to a sink. When the drain of a sink gets "blocked," the water does not drain as quickly, and the water level increases until it overflows. If you can't "unblock" the drain, you need to turn down the water to prevent the sink from overflowing. In the body, the kidneys and liver act as the "drain" when it comes to removing medications from the body. The drain becomes more "blocked" as we age, and, therefore, at the same dose, medication levels in the blood may be higher in older people. Just as you can turn down the water in the sink to prevent it from overflowing, doctors and other healthcare providers can prevent medication levels from getting too high by using lower doses of medications. High levels of medications in the blood can lead to side effects, so it is important that the dose in older people be as low as possible.

Certain diseases can also have an effect on how medications are handled in the body. For example, high blood pressure and diabetes (the disease that increases the amount of sugar in the blood) can damage the kidneys, further "blocking the drain." In addition, some medications can reduce the ability of the kidneys or liver to remove medications from the body. These are some reasons why medications may work differently in older people and why they may have different responses to medication.

The use of over-the-counter (OTC) medication

Many older people take OTC medications (those that can be bought without a prescription at the drug store or grocery store). Many of these medications are very helpful in treating mild symptoms. It is important to remember that some OTC medications may not be recommended in the elderly or may have drug interactions with some prescription medications. Many OTC medications should only be used for short-term treatment, so if you are not getting relief from your symptoms, be sure to contact your doctor. Your doctor may be able to treat the symptoms more effectively.

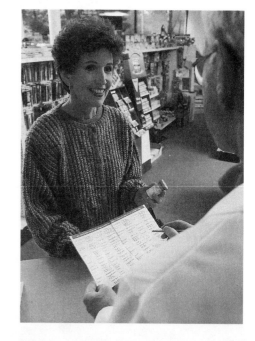

- OTC medications can cause serious side effects. Just like prescription pain medications, some OTC pain medications, such as *Advil®* or *Motrin®* (ibuprofen), *Oruvail®* or *Orudis®* (ketoprofen), or *Aleve®* (naproxen) can cause the kidneys not to work as well ("block the drain") and cause bleeding stomach ulcers (sores). However, used correctly, these pain medications can be safer than their prescription counterparts.

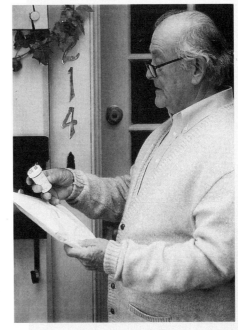

• OTC medications can affect other OTC or prescription medications in many ways. For example, one medication can slow the removal of another medication from the body. This can lead to high blood levels of the other medications which could cause side effects. For example, *Tagamet*® (cimetidine) can slow the removal of an antibiotic such as erythromycin. Some antacids taken to relieve heartburn can block other medications from being absorbed in the stomach. In this case, the other medication will not get into the bloodstream and will not be able to do what it is supposed to do.

• OTC medications can affect how well a disease is controlled. For example, certain medications can cause someone with high blood pressure to have even higher blood pressure. Some examples include *Motrin*®, *Advil*®, etc. (nonsteroidal anti-inflammatory medications) and cold preparations, including phenylpropanolamine.

For these reasons, it is important to talk with your doctor or pharmacist when you are thinking about using an OTC medication, especially if you take a lot of prescription medications. They can even help you pick the best OTC medication for your symptoms. When you visit your doctor or pharmacist, be sure to tell them about any OTC medications you use. They will keep records of the OTC medications you use and let you know if the OTC medication could be a problem. Also, tell your doctor about natural, herbal, or alternative medications. These can also interact with prescription medications.

The effect of aging and disease on taking medication

Changes in the body because of normal aging and some diseases can affect how easily you are able to take your medications. Because close-up vision becomes worse as people age, it may be hard to see the label on your medication bottle and to read the directions easily. Perhaps you cannot read the small writing on the medication information booklets your pharmacist gives you. Be sure to tell your pharmacist if you have vision problems. Be sure to use your reading glasses when taking your medications to prevent errors. If you have trouble reading, talk to your doctor about getting an eye appointment.

Arthritis (stiff, painful joints) is a common problem among older people. If a person's hands are stiff, sore, or weak, he or she might have problems removing the caps from medication bottles or using such things as inhalers (used to breath in medications through the mouth) or syringes (used to give medication through a needle). If you are having problems using your medication, let your pharmacist know. He or she can give you caps that are easier to open and tips for making use of your medication easier.

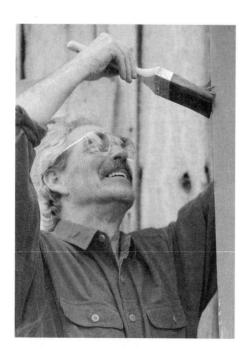

Many older people have changes in their memory as they grow older. Just as it may be hard to remember the name of a person you just met, it may be hard to remember if you took your morning doses of your medication. Memory change is a normal part of aging and is not a cause for worry in most cases. Some medication schedules are harder to remember than others. For example, the instructions for some medications are to take them three times a day. It is often easier for people to take a medication once or twice a day instead of three or four times a day. If you are having problems remembering to take your medications, let your pharmacist or doctor know. Many times it is possible to change to a medication that doesn't need to be taken so often.

It is a good idea to have a special way to help you remember to take your medications. Some people keep their medication bottles on the dining room table, and this reminds them to take their medications whenever they sit down for a meal. Be sure to keep all medications out of the reach of children, however. Some people find it helpful to use a medication pill box in which you can keep all your doses of medications for a whole week at one time. This way, you can look in the box and see if you have taken your medication. There are also several types of "medication reminder systems." Some have an alarm built in that you can set to go off when it's time to take your medication. Your pharmacist can help you find a medication reminder system that is right for you.

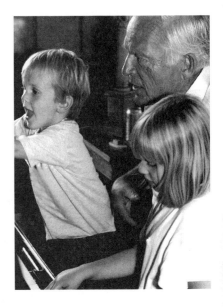

Another problem older people may have is swallowing certain pills. Some medications may be extra large or bitter tasting and may not be pleasant to take. Many times the pharmacist can make it easier for you to take your medication by finding a smaller tablet size, splitting the pills in half, or giving you a liquid form of the medication if it is available.

What you need to know about every medication

There is important information you should know about all of your medications. Your doctor and pharmacist will be able to answer any questions you might have about your medications. Some people may not want to ask questions because they are afraid of looking foolish. Remember, part of the job of a pharmacist or doctor is to make sure that you understand everything you need to know so you can take your medications safely. In the eyes of your doctor and pharmacist, there is no such thing as a "foolish" question when it comes to your health and medications. For people who are taking many medications, it is often helpful to write down this information for each medication on a separate piece of paper. Questions you need answers to include:

- *What is the name of the medication?*

- *Why am I taking this medication? How will I know if it is working? How long do I have to take it?*

- *How do I take this medication? How many times a day? Is it okay to take it with food or are there special instructions? (Some medications cannot be taken with food or certain beverages because the food or drink will block the medication from passing through the stomach into the blood.)*

- *What are the possible side effects? What do I do if I start having a side effect?*

- *What do I do if I miss a dose of the medication?*

- *Are there some medications that I should not use while I am taking this medication?*

- *How should I store this medication? Some medications need to be kept in the refrigerator. It is important to keep other medications in a cool, dry place. Keeping medications in the bathroom cabinet is usually not a good idea because the bathroom is often warm and humid, which can change the effect of the medications.*

Tips for proper medication use

The tips below will help you use your medications safely and will help prevent problems with your medications.

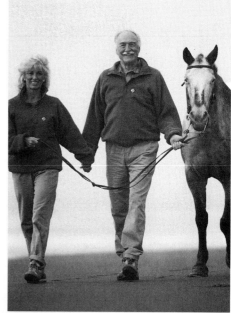

- *Know the side effects that are possible for each of your medications. Contact your pharmacist or doctor if you think you are having a side effect.*

- *Some side effects may show up differently in older people. For example, some medications may make it easier for people to fall or to become confused. If your health changes, remember that it could be due to a side effect. Tell your doctor or pharmacist.*

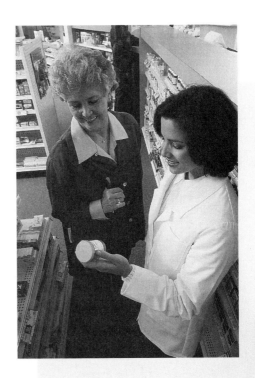

- *Always carry a complete list of all prescription and OTC medications you are taking. You should show this list to all healthcare providers.*

- *Always tell your doctor and pharmacist if you are allergic to any medications.*

- *Throw out all old medications (any medication that has expired or is older than one year).*

- *Never share your medication with anyone else. Sometimes a symptom you have may seem just like what your friend had, but it could be caused by something totally different. It is dangerous to share your medication or to take another person's medication. The dose and the medication were chosen for you; it may be wrong for someone else.*

- *Discuss the use of any over-the-counter or homeopathic (alternative) medication with your doctor and pharmacist before you use it. Some of these medications can cause serious health problems, including unwanted effects that can occur when they are taken along with other medications.*

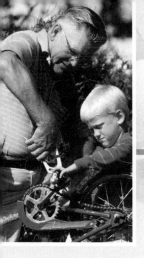

Arthritis and Pain

What are arthritis and pain?

Arthritis

A common cause of pain for older people is arthritis. Arthritis is inflammation (seen as pain, redness, and swelling) of the joints. Over 50% of people past the age of 65 have arthritis. Osteoarthritis is the most common type of arthritis affecting older adults and is caused by wear and tear on the joints. Osteoarthritis most often occurs in knees and hips.

Rheumatoid arthritis is a less common type of arthritis and is thought to be caused by a weakened immune system. While rheumatoid arthritis may occur in older adults, it usually occurs in younger individuals. Arthritis causes pain and sometimes inflammation. Arthritis is painful and may result in swelling and knotting of the joints.

Arthritis can be treated with specific exercises, physical therapy, and medications.

Pain

Pain is an unpleasant feeling or sensation. Pain is usually a sign that part of the body is damaged or injured. Pain can come from injury, inflammation, infection, pressure on tissues, and various other sources. It may be acute (sudden and short-lived) or chronic (long-lasting). Pain may be mild or severe, and each person tolerates pain differently. Pain impulses usually start from the nerve endings in the skin, joints, muscles, or organs that are injured. Next, the pain signals travel along nerves to pain receptors in the brain. The brain senses the pain and sends messages to different parts of the body.

Pain is treated either by blocking receptors in the brain (sites that receive pain signals) or by blocking pain signals that travel from the nerves where the pain starts. Narcotics appear to work on receptors in the brain. Aspirin and related medications (salicylates), acetaminophen, and nonsteroidal anti-inflammatory medications (NSAIDs) probably work by blocking the pain signals that travel to the brain.

Remember that feeling pain is not "normal" for older people. If you have pain that lasts for more than a week or so, talk with your doctor. Doctors help people find out what is causing the pain, and try to remove its cause or treat the pain.

Medications used to treat muscle and joint pain

Tylenol®, *Panadol®*, etc. (acetaminophen), nonsteroidal anti-inflammatory medications (NSAIDs), and salicylates are often used to control the pain of osteoarthritis. Many of the medications used to treat osteoarthritis are also used for rheumatoid arthritis and are listed below. Some medications used for rheumatoid arthritis are not used for osteoarthritis and will not be reviewed in this chapter (i.e., chloroquine, gold, etc.).

Acetaminophen

Acetaminophen is effective for the treatment of mild to moderate aches and pains. It does not irritate the stomach. Due to its lack of side effects and its effectiveness in managing pain, acetaminophen is often the first drug choice in the management of osteoarthritis. Acetaminophen does not reduce inflammation, but it is useful in relieving pain caused by inflammation and osteoarthritis.

Brand Name
Anacin® Aspirin Free
Genapap®
Panadol®
Panex®
St. Joseph's® (Children's Preparation)
Tylenol®
Tylenol® Extra Strength
Tylenol® Regular Strength

How do I use acetaminophen?

Acetaminophen is taken as a tablet, capsule, suppository, or syrup from one to six times a day. It may be taken with or without food and generally does not interfere with other medications. You should not take more than 4000 milligrams a day.

If you miss a dose, don't be concerned. Take your next scheduled dose as needed. Do not double your dose.

What side effects are possible from the use of acetaminophen?

Rare

- allergic reaction
- liver damage

Tell your doctor if you have side effects that do not go away over time, are bothersome, or stop you from taking your medication as directed.

Do other medications interact with acetaminophen?

- Acetaminophen may _decrease_ the effects of _Lamictal_® (lamotrigine).

- Acetaminophen may _decrease_ the effects of _Retrovir_® (zidovudine).

- Acetaminophen may _increase_ the effects of _Coumadin_® (warfarin).

 # Warning

- If an accidental overdose occurs, see a doctor immediately.

- Alcohol (beer, wine, whiskey, etc.) increases your chance of liver damage. If you drink alcohol , you should limit your acetaminophen to no more than 2000 mg daily.

- If you are taking the blood thinner _Coumadin_® (warfarin), you should talk to your doctor before taking acetaminophen.

Nonsteroidal Anti-inflammatory Medications (NSAIDs)

NSAIDs relieve pain and reduce inflammation. These medications are believed to work by preventing the production of prostaglandins, which are chemicals that cause inflammation. They have fewer serious side effects than the steroid preparations and are prescribed more often.

As a group, NSAIDs are similar in the way they work and the side effects they cause. Some, such as _Feldene_® (piroxicam), are longer acting and only need to be taken once a day; others, such as _Motrin_® and _Advil_® (ibuprofen), are short-acting and must be taken more often; some, such as _Butazolidin_® (phenylbutazone), have more powerful anti-inflammatory effects, but more side effects as well.

"▲" Indicates medications that are <u>generally not recommended</u> for use in older people. Do not stop taking these medications unless directed by your doctor. They may be required under special circumstances. Talk to your doctor to see if this medication is right for you.

Brand Name	Generic
▲ *Butazolidin®*	phenylbutazone
▲ *Indocin®*	indomethacin
Advil®	ibuprofen
Aleve®	naproxen
Anaprox®	naproxen
Ansaid®	flurbiprofen
Clinoril®	sulindac
Daypro®	oxaprozin
Duract®	bromfenac
Feldene®	piroxicam
Lodine®	etodolac
Meclomen®	meclofenamate
Motrin®	ibuprofen
Nalfon®	fenoprofen
Naprosyn®	naproxen

Chart continues on next page

Brand Name	Generic
Orudis®	ketoprofen
Oruvail®	ketoprofen
Ponstel®	mefenamic acid
Relafen®	nabumetone
Tolectin®	tolmetin
Toradol®	ketorolac
Voltaren®	diclofenac

If one NSAID does not work for you, this does not mean that a different NSAID will not work. Your doctor may prescribe several different NSAIDs before finding the one that best fits your needs. Some may cause you less stomach upset. But there is no advantage to taking smaller doses of two different NSAIDs instead of an effective dose of one.

How do I use NSAIDs?

These medications are prescribed from one to four times per day depending on which NSAID you take. Because they commonly cause stomach upset, such as nausea, vomiting, or stomach pain, and can cause ulcers, it is best to take them with food, milk, or an antacid. The pain-relieving effect will usually start within one hour; however, it may take up to one or more weeks to get the full anti-inflammatory effect.

If you miss a dose, don't be concerned. Take your next scheduled dose as needed. Do not double your dose.

What side effects are possible from the use of NSAIDs?

More Common

- nausea or vomiting
- constipation
- diarrhea

Less Common

- headache
- kidney problems with water retention and swelling
- ringing in the ears (tinnitus) or hearing loss
- skin rash
- stomach ulcers/bleeding

Rare

- itching
- confusion/dizziness/drowsiness, especially with *Indocin*® (indomethacin)
- depression (sadness that doesn't go away)
- heartburn
- behavioral changes
- blurred vision
- loss of sense of taste or altered sense of taste
- rapid heartbeat and palpitations
- kidney or liver failure
- life-threatening bleeding
- bone marrow failure with anemia and weakening of the immune system, especially with *Butazolidin*® (phenylbutazone)

Tell your doctor if you have side effects that do not go away over time, are bothersome, or stop you from taking your medication as directed.

Do other medications interact with NSAIDs?

- NSAIDs may have _increased_ side effects with over-the-counter (OTC) medications that contain aspirin or other NSAIDs. Many OTC pain and cold medications contain pain relievers, and the names are confusing. Talk to your doctor or pharmacist before taking any OTC medications.

- NSAIDs may _increase_ the effects of anticoagulants (blood thinners) like Coumadin® (warfarin) by increasing the blood-thinning effect and increasing the chance of a bleeding ulcer.

- NSAIDs may _decrease_ the blood pressure-lowering effects of blood pressure medication.

- NSAIDs may _decrease_ the effects of diuretics (water pills).

- NSAIDs may _increase_ the effects of methotrexate.

- NSAIDs may _increase_ the effects of Dilantin® (phenytoin).

- Benemid® (probenecid) may _increase_ the effects of NSAIDs.

 Warning

- Allergic reactions may produce a skin rash, wheezing, and difficulty in breathing. Such reactions are most likely to occur in people with a known sensitivity to aspirin. If you have had a previous reaction to aspirin or any other anti-inflammatory medication, avoid NSAIDs entirely.

- Stomach pain may be a sign of an ulcer. If ulcers are left untreated, they may cause serious bleeding. Tell your doctor if you have stomach pain that is severe or keeps returning, or if you have a history of peptic ulcer disease. Call your doctor immediately if you notice dark, coffee-ground-looking stools or if you are vomiting dark material that looks like coffee grounds. These may be signs of a bleeding ulcer.

- People with kidney disease, liver disease, or congestive heart failure may have worsening of these illnesses with NSAIDs. Be sure to tell your doctor if you have these conditions. If you have these conditions, talk to your doctor before taking any OTC medications, since NSAIDs are in many OTC medications.

- NSAIDs affect the function of platelets (the cells partly responsible for blood clotting) and should be stopped two to three days prior to surgery.

- *Butazolidin®* (phenylbutazone) can cause serious damage to the bone marrow. It is not generally recommended for use in older patients because safer medications are available. If you are taking *Butazolidin®*, talk to your doctor to see if it is the right medication for you. Do not stop taking the medication without speaking to your doctor.

- *Indocin®* (indomethacin) can cause light-headedness and confusion. It is not recommended for use in older patients because safer medications are available. If you are taking *Indocin®*, talk to your doctor to see if it is the right drug for you. Do not stop taking the medication without speaking to your doctor.

Salicylates (Aspirin and Aspirin-Like Compounds)

Aspirin and the other salicylates are among the most commonly used anti-inflammatory agents.

Like other NSAIDs, these can relieve pain, reduce inflammation, and control fever. In order to reduce inflammation, salicylates must be taken in larger doses than would be necessary to relieve pain or control fever. The right dose must be decided for each person, and some people may require up to 12 aspirin tablets per day. Higher doses are used for rheumatoid arthritis than for osteoarthritis.

Brand Name	Generic
Arthritis Pain Formula®	aspirin
Ascriptin®	aspirin
Bayer® Aspirin (regular strength)	aspirin
Bayer® Aspirin Maximum Strength	aspirin
Bayer® Children's Aspirin	aspirin
Bayer® Enteric-Coated	aspirin
Bufferin®	aspirin
Disalcid®	salsalate
Dolobid®	diflunisal
Ecotrin®	aspirin
Empirin®	aspirin
Halfprin®	aspirin
Magan®	magnesium salicylate
Mobidin®	magnesium salicylate
Trilisate®	choline magnesium salicylates
various	choline magnesium

How do I use salicylates (aspirin and aspirin-like compounds)?

Most salicylates are taken several times a day, usually with food or an antacid, because they can cause stomach upset. A number of types are coated or combined with buffers to be less damaging to the stomach. They may reduce some of the symptoms but do not remove all the side effects. Do not crush or chew the pills. Take the medication with a full 8-ounce glass of water to prevent pills from sticking in your throat.

If you miss a dose, don't be concerned. Take your next scheduled dose as needed. Do not double your dose.

What side effects are possible from the use of salicylates?

More Common

- nausea or vomiting
- heartburn

Less Common

- ringing in the ears (tinnitus) or hearing loss
- stomach ulcers/bleeding
- iron deficient anemia
- bruising

Rare

- allergic reactions: skin rash, hives, itching, angioedema (swelling of face and throat)
- shortness of breath
- life-threatening bleeding
- salicylism: dizziness, diarrhea, confusion, headache, sweating, hyperventilation (fast, troubled breathing)

Tell your doctor if you have side effects that do not go away over time, are bothersome, or stop you from taking your medication as directed.

Do other medications interact with aspirin?

Aspirin may *increase* the effects of the following medications:

- anticoagulants (blood thinners)

- *Depakote*®, *Depakene*® (valproic acid)

- *Rheumatrex*® (methotrexate)

Aspirin may _decrease_ the effects of the following medications:

- _Anturane®_ (sulfinpyrazone)
- _Benemid®_ (probenecid)
- blood pressure medications
- diuretics (water pills)

 # Warning

- Aspirin should not be used by children (under 18 years of age) because it may cause Reye's syndrome, a life-threatening condition that can lead to coma and death. Keep this and all medications away from small children.

Narcotics and Narcotic-Like Agents

Narcotics work on receptors (sites that receive pain signals) in the brain to relieve pain. They may also cause drowsiness, confusion, and constipation. Narcotics are powerful pain relievers and should be used only when pain is severe because they cause many side effects in older people and can be addicting (feeling that you can't stop taking the drug). However, in patients who are dying of cancer or other life-ending conditions that cause lasting pain, narcotics should be used in high enough doses to relieve pain and make the patient comfortable. In these cases, side effects and addiction are not a large concern.

Single-agent medications:

"▲" Indicates medications that are generally not recommended for use in older people. Do not stop taking these medications unless directed by your doctor. They may be required under special circumstances. Talk to your doctor to see if this medication is right for you.

Brand Name	Generic
▲ Darvon®	propoxyphene
▲ Demerol®	meperidine
▲ Talwin®	pentazocine
Dilaudid®	hydromorphone
M S Contin®	morphine
Stadol®	butorphanol
various	codeine

Combination medications:

narcotics + aspirin (ASA) or narcotics + acetaminophen (APAP)

Brand Name	Generic
▲ Darvocet N®	propoxyphene & APAP
▲ Darvon® Compound-65	propoxyphene & ASA
▲ Talacen®	pentazocine & APAP
▲ Talwin® Compound	pentazocine & ASA
▲ Wygesic®	propoxyphene & APAP
Lortab®	hydrocodone & APAP
Percocet®	oxycodone & APAP
Percodan®	oxycodone & ASA
Phenaphen® with Codeine	codeine & APAP
Tylenol® with Codeine	codeine & APAP
Vicodin®	hydrocodone & APAP

How do I use narcotics and narcotic-like agents?

Narcotics come in the form of pills, syrups, suppositories, or injections. They should be taken exactly the way they are prescribed by your doctor. They are generally not affected by food. Most older people need to take a stimulant laxative to prevent constipation when using narcotics. Talk to your doctor or pharmacist for advice about laxatives you can use safely.

If you miss a dose, don't be concerned. Take your next scheduled dose as needed. Do not double your dose.

What side effects are possible from the use of narcotics?

More Common

- loss of appetite
- constipation
- nausea
- small pupils
- drowsiness
- difficulty urinating

Less Common

- vomiting
- confusion, dizziness
- slowed pulse and breathing
- flushing
- low blood pressure
- itching

Tell your doctor if you have side effects that do not go away over time, are bothersome, or stop you from taking your medication as directed.

Do other medications interact with narcotics?

- The effects of narcotics are increased when taken with other medications that cause drowsiness, such as antipsychotic medications, barbiturates, antianxiety medications, sleeping pills, or antihistamines. Talk to your doctor or pharmacist before taking any over-the-counter medications because they may also increase the side effects of narcotics.

- People taking MAO inhibitors such as *Nardil*® (phenelzine) or *Parnate*® (tranylcypromine) must not take narcotics; the combination can be deadly. It is important to tell your doctor if you are taking any other medications.

- *Darvon*®, *Darvocet*®, and *Wygesic*® (all are the brand names of propoxyphene) may <u>increase</u> the effects of *Tegretol*® (carbamazepine) and *Coumadin*® (warfarin).

- *Dilantin*® (phenytoin) may <u>increase</u> the effects of *Demerol*® (meperidine).

What else are narcotics used for?

Occasionally, morphine is used to control an episode of severe heart failure or a heart attack. Narcotics are also used to quiet coughing.

 # Warning

- *Darvon*®, *Darvon*® Compound-65, *Darvocet*®, or *Wygesic*® (propoxyphene) are no stronger than *Tylenol*® (acetaminophen) for relieving pain, but causes the same side effects as other narcotics. This medication should be avoided by older patients. If you are taking propoxyphene, talk to your doctor to see if it is the right medication for you. Do not stop taking the medication without speaking with your doctor.

- *Talwin*® (pentazocine) is an effective narcotic, but it tends to cause confusion and nightmares. Older patients should avoid this medication. If you are taking *Talwin*®, talk with your doctor to see if it is the right medication for you. Do not stop taking the medication without speaking to your doctor.

- *Demerol®* (meperidine) is not a very effective pain reliever, and the drug can build up in older people, causing serious side effects such as seizures. This drug should be avoided in older people. If you are taking *Demerol®*, talk with your doctor to see if it is the right drug for you. Do not stop taking the medication without speaking to your doctor.

- Narcotics can affect one's ability to breathe. Tell your doctor if you have asthma, emphysema, bronchitis, or other lung diseases.

- Narcotics can cause drowsiness and interfere with mental functioning. Avoid operating machinery, driving, or performing other possibly dangerous tasks that require alertness. Never drink alcohol (beer, wine, whiskey, etc.) while taking narcotics.

- Combination narcotics with aspirin or acetaminophen may have increased side effects with over-the-counter (OTC) medications that contain aspirin, nonsteroidal anti-inflammatory medications (NSAIDs), or *Tylenol®* (acetaminophen). Many OTC pain and cold medications contain pain relievers. Talk to your doctor or pharmacist before taking any OTC medications.

- If you have been taking narcotics for a long time, stopping the medication suddenly without slowly lowering the dose under your doctor's guidance may cause withdrawal symptoms such as sweating, flushing, twitching, tremors, and irritability.

Ultram® (tramadol)

Ultram® is not a narcotic but works at receptors. It is used for moderate to severe pain.

How do I use Ultram®?

Ultram® is taken every four to six hours as needed for pain.

If you miss a dose, don't be concerned. Take your next scheduled dose as needed. Do not double your dose.

What side effects are possible from the use of Ultram®?

- dizziness, drowsiness
- nausea, vomiting, heartburn
- diarrhea
- constipation
- vertigo (balance problems)
- itching
- sweating
- dry mouth

Tell your doctor if you have side effects that do not go away over time, are bothersome, or stop you from taking your medication as directed.

Do other medications interact with Ultram®?

- Do not use *Ultram®* (tramadol) with *Nardil®* or *Parnate®* (MAO inhibitors).

- *Tegretol®* (carbamazepine) can <u>decrease</u> the effectiveness of *Ultram®* (tramadol).

 # Warning

- *Ultram®* can cause drowsiness and interfere with alert mental functioning. Avoid operating machinery, driving, or performing other possibly dangerous tasks that require alertness. Do not drink alcohol (beer, wine, whiskey, etc.) while using this medication.

- *Ultram®* can build up in patients with kidney or liver disease and cause side effects. Tell your doctor if you have any kidney or liver problems.

- While *Ultram®* is not a narcotic, dependence on it (the feeling that you always need the medication) can develop. To avoid dependence, take it only as prescribed by your doctor.

Corticosteroids

Among the most powerful medications to reduce inflammation are the corticosteroids. They are sometimes used in treatment of rheumatoid arthritis but are usually saved for severe diseases.

Brand Name	Generic
Aristocort®	triamcinolone
Celestone®	betamethasone
Cortef®	hydrocortisone
Decadron®	dexamethasone
Delta-Cortef®	prednisolone
Deltasone®	prednisone
Hexadrol®	dexamethasone
Medrol®	methylprednisolone
Orasone®	prednisone
various	cortisone

How do I use corticosteroids?

They may be taken by mouth, intravenously, rectally, or by injection into an affected joint (intra-articular injection). Injections are extremely useful if only a few joints are involved. Oral corticosteroids may be taken one to several times a day. It is best to take them with food or antacids to reduce the chance of stomach upset. To prevent unnecessary side effects, the doctor will prescribe the lowest dose possible to reduce your symptoms. Do not increase your dose without talking with your doctor.

If you miss a dose of this medication, take it as soon as possible. However, if it is almost time for your next dose, skip the missed dose and go back to the dosing schedule. Do not double your dose. It is very important to take your medication exactly as directed by your doctor. NEVER stop taking your prescription medications without talking with your doctor.

What side effects are possible from the use of corticosteroids?

- osteoporosis (fragile bones)
- worsening or unmasking diabetes
- cataracts, glaucoma
- increased chance of infection
- mood swings, psychosis (strange behavior) from high doses
- easy bruising, thinning of the skin, broken blood vessels
- upset stomach, ulcers
- fluid buildup and swelling
- worsening high blood pressure

Tell your doctor if you have side effects that do not go away over time, are bothersome, or stop you from taking your medication as directed.

Do other medications interact with corticosteroids?

Corticosteroid effects may <u>decrease</u> when taken with the following:

- *Dilantin®* (phenytoin)
- *Rifadin®* (rifampin)
- barbiturates

Corticosteroid effects may <u>increase</u> when taken with the following:

- *Premarin®, Ogen®* (estrogens)
- *Nizoral®* (ketoconazole)
- *Ery-tabs®, PCE®* (erythromycin)

Doses of oral hypoglycemics, insulin, potassium supplements, and diuretics may need to be increased when taking corticosteroids.

Corticosteroids may <u>increase</u> the effects of *Lanoxin®* (digoxin).

What else can corticosteroids be used for?

Corticosteroids can be used in other diseases that cause inflammation (incidences of acute gout, asthma, etc.) or when other anti-inflammatory medications are not working or not recommended. They are also used to stop the body's defense system from attacking the body itself, which occurs with several conditions called autoimmune diseases.

 # Warning

- Blood levels of glucose and electrolytes (especially potassium) should be checked regularly in diabetics and in people taking diuretics (water pills).

- Corticosteroids can mask symptoms of an infection and can decrease the body's defense against infection. Call your doctor if you have a lasting cough, fever, or sore throat.

- Cataracts and glaucoma can develop with long-term corticosteroid use.

- Stopping the medication suddenly without slowly lowering the dose may cause withdrawal symptoms like nausea, decreased appetite, difficulty breathing, low blood pressure, low blood sugar, muscle pain, and fainting. Do not stop taking this medication without talking to your doctor.

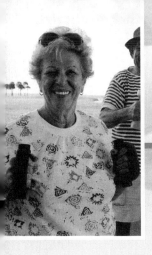

Breathing Problems

What are breathing problems (asthma, emphysema, and chronic bronchitis)?

A breathing disorder is a condition that occurs when the airways in the lungs are blocked, limiting the amount of air that can get through. Asthma, emphysema, and chronic bronchitis are some of the more common types of this disorder that occur in older people. Emphysema and chronic bronchitis are often called chronic obstructive pulmonary disease (COPD). They are usually closely related to smoking. Symptoms include chronic coughing and shortness of breath. In emphysema, the small airways have collapsed, so they restrict the flow of air. In chronic bronchitis, the airways are inflamed, swollen, and blocked with mucus.

People with asthma have extra-sensitive airways that narrow when triggered by certain things, such as allergies, air pollution, stress, and infections. Symptoms include wheezing, coughing, a feeling of tightness in the chest, and shortness of breath.

Treatment for these conditions may include medications, quitting smoking or limiting exposure to other people's smoke, and daily exercise.

Medications used to treat breathing problems

Beta-Adrenergic Bronchodilators (Beta-Agonists)

Beta-adrenergic bronchodilators relax the muscles surrounding the airways. This opens the airways, allowing air to pass more easily into the lungs. They also help to clear extra mucus (phlegm).

Brand Name	Generic
Adrenalin®	epinephrine
Alupent®	metaproterenol
AsthmaHaler® Mist	epinephrine
AsthmaNefrin®	epinephrine
Brethaire®	terbutaline
Brethine®	terbutaline
Bricanyl®	terbutaline
Bronkaid Mist®	epinephrine
Bronkometer®	isoetharine mesylate
Bronkosol®	isoetharine
Dispos-a-Med®	isuprel
Duo-Medihaler®	isoproterenol/phenylephrine
Maxair®	pirbuterol
Medihaler-Iso®	isoproterenol
Metaprel®	metaproterenol
Proventil®	albuterol
Serevent®	salmeterol
Sus-Phrine®	epinephrine
Tornalate®	bitolterol
Ventolin®	albuterol

How do I use beta-adrenergic bronchodilators?

Beta-adrenergic bronchodilators are available in three forms:

1. Metered-Dose Inhaler (MDI): The best way to lessen the symptoms of COPD and asthma is to use an inhalant (a medication that is breathed into the lungs). That is because it delivers the drug directly to the site of the problem – the airways and lungs. Instructions for using MDIs are located at the end of this chapter. Some older people have trouble using inhalers. A number of devices, such as tubes and spacers, can make it easier to use inhalers. Make sure you know exactly how to use your inhaler. Let your doctor or healthcare provider watch you use your inhaler to make sure you are using it correctly.

2. Nebulizer: A liquid form of the medication can be made into a spray mist and inhaled through a machine called a nebulizer. Nebulizers are useful for people who need larger doses than inhalers can provide or who suffer severe acute (sudden) asthma attacks. Nebulizers can also be useful for those who have trouble using inhaler devices (even with a spacer) because of arthritis, stroke, or poor eyesight.

3. Oral Medications: Tablets must contain higher doses of beta-adrenergic bronchodilators than inhalants to be effective, so side effects are more common. Pills also take longer to work. People who cannot use inhalers properly may need to use tablets.

If you miss a dose of this medication, take it as soon as possible. However, if it is almost time for your next dose, skip the missed dose and go back to the dosing schedule. Do not double your dose. It is very important to take your medication exactly as directed by your doctor. NEVER stop taking your prescription medications without talking with your doctor.

What side effects are possible from the use of beta-adrenergic bronchodilators?

More Common

- faster heartbeat
- shakiness and nervousness
- insomnia (trouble sleeping)

Less Common

- headache
- increased blood pressure
- a feeling of increased or irregular heartbeat
- anxiety

Rare

- difficulty urinating/emptying bladder

Side effects are more of a problem with epinephrine, isoproterenol, and oral agents. But side effects may occur with any beta-adrenergic bronchodilator.

Tell your doctor if you have side effects that do not go away over time, are bothersome, or stop you from taking your medication as directed.

Do other medications interact with beta-adrenergic bronchodilators?

- Beta-blockers decrease the effectiveness of the beta-adrenergic bronchodilators.

- *Parnate®* and *Nardil®* (MAO inhibitors) should not be taken in combination with inhaled beta-adrenergic bronchodilators. The combinations may cause severe high blood pressure or death.

What else should I know about beta-adrenergic bronchodilators (beta-agonists)?

• You may experience worsening symptoms, shortness of breath and closing of the airways after overuse (more than 16 puffs a day) of these agents. Use only as directed by your doctor. Notify your doctor if you need more medication than you were prescribed.

• *Serevent®* (salmeterol), a long-acting beta-adrenergic bronchodilator, is indicated for chronic treatment only. It should not be used in *emergency situations*.

 ## Warning

• Beta-adrenergic bronchodilators may cause special problems in some people suffering from heart disease, high blood pressure, or thyroid disease. Be sure your doctor is aware of your full medical history before you use any of these medications.

• Some inhalers are meant for use in *emergency situations* when immediate relief of breathing problems is needed. Others are used every day to prevent symptoms. Make sure you know which inhaler is used for each situation. Ask your doctor or pharmacist if you have any questions.

Theophylline

Theophylline opens the airways, reduces the release of phlegm, and stimulates the breathing center in the brain, the diaphragm (the muscle below the lungs that helps them to draw in air), and the heart. It also helps to get rid of some fluid in the lungs, and increases urination, which is sometimes helpful. Theophylline taken by mouth is usually given for long-term treatment of asthma and chronic obstructive pulmonary disease (COPD).

Brand Name	Generic
Slo-Phyllin®	theophylline
Theobid®	theophylline
Theo-Dur®	theophylline
Theolair-SR®	theophylline

How do I use theophylline ?

Theophylline is usually taken in pill form one to four times a day depending on the type of pill prescribed. Theophylline is also available as a syrup or as a rectal suppository, helpful if one has difficulty swallowing pills. Do not crush or break the sustained-release preparations (long-acting tablets of capsules like *Theo-Dur®*, *Slo-Phyllin®*, etc.).

If you miss a dose of this medication, take it as soon as possible. However, if it is almost time for your next dose, skip the missed dose and go back to the dosing schedule. Do not double your dose. It is very important to take your medication exactly as directed by your doctor. NEVER stop taking your prescription medications without talking with your doctor.

What side effects are possible from the use of theophylline?

More Common

- stomach upset or stomach pain
- dizziness
- nausea
- nervousness
- vomiting
- insomnia (trouble sleeping)

- shakiness
- headache
- stomach pain
- increased urination

Less Common

- palpitations
- rapid or irregular heartbeat
- fever
- agitation ("hyper" feeling)
- high blood sugar
- seizures

Tell your doctor if you have side effects that do not go away over time, are bothersome, or stop you from taking your medication as directed.

Do other medications interact with theophylline?

The following medications may *increase* the effects of theophylline:

Tagamet®(cimetidine), *Premarin*®(estrogens), *Cipro*®(ciprofloxacin), *Zyloprim*®(allopurinol), *Ery-Tab*® and *PCE*® (erythromycin), *TAO*® (troleandomycin), *Inderal*®(propranolol), *Nizoral*®(ketoconazole).

The following conditions may *increase* the effects of theophylline:

congestive heart failure, liver disease, pneumonia/viral infections, and a large increase of carbohydrates in the diet

The following medications may *decrease* the effects of theophylline:

Rifadin®(rifampin), *Luminal*®(phenobarbital), *Dilantin*®(phenytoin), *Tegretol*®(carbamazepine), *Nizoral*®(ketoconazole)

The following conditions may *decrease* the effects of theophylline:

smoking, a significant increase of protein in the diet, and eating charcoal-broiled food

What else should I know about theophylline?

• Be sure to have your theophylline blood levels checked (generally every six months once you are kept on the same dose).

• People with peptic ulcer disease, heart disease, gout, and diabetes mellitus should use theophylline carefully.

• Do not eat or drink large amounts of caffeine-containing products (colas, coffee, chocolate) to avoid the increased chance of side effects.

Anticholinergic Bronchodilators

These medications work by allowing the airways to relax. These agents are more effective in COPD than in asthma.

Brand Name	Generic
Atrovent®	ipratropium bromide
Combivent®	albuterol/ipratropium bromide

How do I use anticholinergic bronchodilators?

Anticholinergic bronchodilators come in two forms:

1. Metered-Dose Inhaler (MDI): The best way to lessen the symptoms of COPD and asthma is to use an inhalant. That is because it delivers the drug directly to the site of the problem – the airways and lungs. Instructions for using MDIs are located at the end of this chapter. Some older people have trouble using inhalers. Special equipment, such as tubes and spacers, can make it easier to use inhalers. Make sure you know exactly how to use your inhaler. Let your doctor or healthcare provider watch you use your inhaler to make sure you are using it correctly.

2. Nebulizer: A liquid form of the medication can be turned into a mist and inhaled through a machine called a nebulizer. Nebulizers are useful for people who require larger doses than inhalers can provide or who suffer severe acute asthma attacks. Nebulizers can also be useful for individuals who have trouble using inhaler devices (even with a spacer) because of arthritis, stroke, or poor eyesight.

If you take a regularly scheduled dose of a beta-agonist in combination with the anticholinergic bronchodilator, take the beta-agonist first and then the anticholinergic bronchodilator.

If you miss a dose of this medication, take it as soon as possible. However, if it is almost time for your next dose, skip the missed dose and go back to the dosing schedule. Do not double your dose. It is very important to take your medication exactly as directed by your doctor. NEVER stop taking your prescription medications without talking with your doctor.

What side effects are possible from the use of anticholinergic bronchodilators?

More Common

- dry mouth
- rapid heartbeat (temporary)
- cough
- nervousness
- dizziness
- headache

Less Common

- difficulty urinating/emptying bladder
- flushing
- blurred vision
- widened pupils in the eye

Tell your doctor if you have side effects that do not go away over time, are bothersome, or stop you from taking your medication as directed.

Do other medications interact with anticholinergic bronchodilators?

Side effects may be made worse if anticholinergic bronchodilators are taken in combination with other medications that have similar effects, such as *Elavil®*, *Sinequan®*, etc. (tricyclic antidepressants), *Thorazine®*, *Stelazine®*, etc. (antipsychotics), and *Benadryl®*, *Chlortrimeton®*, etc. (antihistamines).

 # Warning

- If you have the eye condition glaucoma, use caution to avoid spraying in your eyes.

- If you have difficulty urinating, this medication may make the condition worse.

Corticosteroids

Corticosteroids are a powerful type of the medications called anti-inflammatory medications. As the name suggests, these medications work to reduce inflammation (swelling and irritation). They also decrease phlegm production. Steroids are more effective in asthma than in COPD. The inhaled steroid agents are used for long-term, day-to-day prevention of breathing problems; do not use these medications to treat sudden attacks. Steroids may help decrease the need for regularly scheduled beta-agonists.

Corticosteroids: oral

Brand Name	Generic
Cortef®	hydrocortisone
Cortone®	cortisone
Decadron®	dexamethasone
Delta-Cortef®	prednisolone
Deltasone®	prednisone
Hexadrol®	dexamethasone
Hydrocortone®	hydrocortisone
Medrol®	methylprednisolone
Meticorten®	prednisone
Orasone®	prednisone
Prelone®	prednisolone

Corticosteroids: inhaled

Brand Name	Generic
AeroBid®	flunisolide
Azmacort®	triamcinolone
Beclovent®	beclomethosone
Decadron®	dexamethasone
Decadron® Phosphate	dexamethasone
Flovent®	fluticasone
Respihaler®	dexamethasone
Vanceril®	beclomethasone

How do I use corticosteroids?

1. Metered-Dose Inhaler (MDI): The best way to lessen the symptoms of COPD and asthma is to use an inhalant. That is because it delivers the drug directly to the site of the problem – the airways and lungs. Instructions for using MDIs are located at the end of this chapter. Some older people have trouble using inhalers. A number of devices, such as tubes and reservoir spacers, can make it easier to use inhalers. Make sure you know exactly how to use your inhaler. Let your doctor or healthcare provider watch you use your inhaler to make sure you are using it correctly. *Flovent*® (fluticasone) is also available as a dry-powder inhaler.

If you take a regularly scheduled dose of a beta-agonist in combination with the corticosteroid, take the beta-agonist first and then the corticosteroid inhaler.

The inhaled steroid preparations cause side effects less often. If you also use a beta-agonist inhaler, it is generally best to use your steroid inhaler about 5 to 15 minutes after the beta-agonist to allow the medication to penetrate deeper into the lungs. Rinse mouth after inhaling.

2. Oral Medications: Pills must contain higher doses of the corticosteroid than inhalants to be effective, so side effects are more common. Pills also take longer to work. People who cannot use inhalants properly may need to use pills. People with worsening conditions may also need pills.

The oral preparations (usually prednisone) are generally taken once a day in the morning. It may be recommended that you take the medication every other day instead to decrease side effects if steroids are to be used on a long-term basis. Take steroids with food to avoid stomach irritation.

If you miss a dose of this medication, take it as soon as possible. However, if it is almost time for your next dose, skip the missed dose and go back to the dosing schedule. Do not double your dose. It is very important to take your medication exactly as directed by your doctor. NEVER stop taking your prescription medications without talking with your doctor.

What side effects are possible from the use of oral steroids?

Steroids have many side effects, especially if used for a long period of time.

Short-term therapy:

More Common

- stomach upset
- stomach irritation or ulcers
- increased risk of infections
- swelling of the hands, feet, face
- low potassium
- mood swings
- worsening of diabetes (increased blood sugar)
- increased appetite

Long-term therapy:

More Common

- osteoporosis (thin, weak bones)
- acne
- muscle weakness
- hair growth
- cataracts
- weight gain
- increase in blood pressure
- easy bruising
- worsening of glaucoma (an eye disease)

What else can oral steroids be used for?

Oral steroids can also be used for the treatment of arthritis (and related diseases), allergies, skin conditions, chronic liver diseases, blood disorders, kidney diseases, and inflammatory conditions, such as gout or bursitis.

Inhaled Steroids

What side effects are possible from the use of inhaled steroids?

More Common

- oral thrush (yeast infection of the mouth)
- coughing and wheezing (on use)
- sore throat
- dry mouth
- hoarseness or voice changes

Tell your doctor if you have side effects that do not go away over time, are bothersome, or stop you from taking your medication as directed.

Do other medications interact with corticosteroids?

The following medications may *increase* the effects of corticosteroids:

- *Premarin*® (estrogens)
- *Nizoral*® (ketoconazole)
- *Erytabs*®, *PCE*® (erythromycin)

The following medications may _decrease_ the effects of corticosteroids:

- _Dilantin®_ (phenytoin)
- _Rifadin®_ (rifampin)
- barbiturates

Corticosteroids, when taken with some nonsteroidal anti-inflammatory medications, may increase the risk of ulcers in the stomach and intestines.

Doses of insulin or oral diabetes medications, diuretics (water pills), potassium supplements, or blood pressure medications may need to be adjusted when taking steroids.

Corticosteroids may increase the effects of _Lanoxin®_ (digoxin).

What else should I know about corticosteroids?

- After each use of the steroid MDI, rinse your mouth well with water or mouthwash to help prevent throat infections.

- These medications are to be taken on a regular schedule, though the benefits may not be seen for several weeks.

- Wear a MedicAlert bracelet stating that you use steroids.

- Long-term use of steroids may weaken the body's ability to fight infection and the effects of stress.

- Before taking steroids, tell your doctor if you have had tuberculosis or ulcer disease in the past, or if you have diabetes or high blood pressure.

- Be sure that all of your doctors know that you are taking steroids.

- If you are on steroids for a long time, tell your doctor immediately if you think that you are getting an infection while taking steroids. Some signs of infection include fever, chills, sore throat and redness, soreness, and/or swelling around a cut or other injury to the skin.

- Inhaled steroids are for long-term prevention. They are not meant for emergency use when immediate relief of breathing problems is needed.

 # Warning

- If you have taken oral steroid medications for more than a few days, never stop taking them all at once. Doing so can cause death. It is very important to lower the dose of steroids slowly. NEVER SUDDENLY DISCONTINUE ORAL STEROIDS EXCEPT ON YOUR DOCTOR'S ADVICE.

- Some inhalers are meant for use in *emergency situations* when immediate relief of breathing problems is needed. Others are used every day to prevent symptoms. Make sure you know which inhaler is used for each situation. Ask your doctor or pharmacist if you have any questions.

Intal® (Cromolyn Sodium) and Tilade® (Nedocromil Sodium)

Intal® and *Tilade®* prevent the release of allergic-type substances within the lungs. These are useful for long-term asthma, especially asthma caused by exercise or cold air.

Brand Name	Generic
Intal®	cromolyn sodium
Tilade®	nedocromil sodium

How do I use Intal®?

Intal® or *Tilade®* is taken by an MDI on a regular schedule, usually two puffs, four times a day. You may also be told to take two puffs at least 10 to 15 minutes before exercising or going out into cold weather. It may take up to four weeks to see the greatest benefits from cromolyn or nedocromil.

1. Metered-Dose Inhaler (MDI): The best way to lessen the symptoms of chronic asthma is to use an inhalant. That is because the MDI delivers the drug directly to the site of the problem – the airway and lungs. Instructions for using MDIs are located at the end of this chapter. Some older people have trouble using inhalers. Special equipment, such as tubes and reservoir spacers, can make it easier to use inhalers. Make sure you know exactly how to use your inhaler. Let your doctor or healthcare provider watch you use your inhaler to make sure you are using it correctly.

2. Nebulizer: A liquid form of the medication can be made into a spray mist and inhaled through a machine called a nebulizer. Nebulizers are useful for people who need larger doses than inhalers can provide or who suffer severe sudden asthma attacks. Nebulizers can also be useful for individuals who have trouble using inhalers (even with a spacer) because of arthritis, stroke, or poor eyesight.

If you miss a dose of this medication, take it as soon as possible. However, if it is almost time for your next dose, skip the missed dose and go back to the dosing schedule. Do not double your dose. It is very important to take your medication exactly as directed by your doctor. NEVER stop taking your prescription medications without talking with your doctor.

What side effects are possible from the use of Intal® or Tilade®?

Intal® or *Tilade®* causes no problem side effects in most people. You may experience a temporary unpleasant taste or hoarseness. It will go away.

Tell your doctor if you have side effects that do not go away over time, are bothersome, or stop you from taking your medication as directed.

Warning

- People with irregular heartbeats, or liver, kidney, or heart disease should be careful when taking this medication. Be sure your doctor knows your full medical history before you use any of these medications.

- Some medications are meant for use in *emergency situations when immediate relief of breathing problems is needed.* Others are used every day to prevent symptoms. Make sure you know which inhaler is used for each situation. Ask your doctor or pharmacist if you have any questions.

- This medication should not be used for *emergency situations when immediate relief from breathing problems is needed.*

Leukotriene Antagonists

These medications are used to treat asthma. They help prevent the airways from swelling and blocking airflow and decrease mucus production.

Brand Name	Generic
Accolate®	zafirlukast
Singulair®	montelukast sodium
Zyflo®	zileuton

How do I use leukotriene antagonists?

These medications are pills taken by mouth, usually one, two or four times a day. They should be taken every day and are for continuous use. *Accolate®* (zafirlukast) and *Zyflo®* (zileuton) should be taken one hour before meals or two hours after meals. *Singulair®* (montelukast) should be taken in the evening with or without food.

If you miss a dose of this medication, take it as soon as possible. However, if it is almost time for your next dose, skip the missed dose and go back to the dosing schedule. Do not double your dose. It is very important to take your medication exactly as directed by your doctor. NEVER stop taking your prescription medications without talking with your doctor.

What side effects are possible from the use of leukotriene antagonists?

More Common

- headache

Less Common

- diarrhea
- dizziness

Rare

- liver problems

Tell your doctor if you have side effects that do not go away over time, are bothersome, or stop you from taking your medication as directed.

Do other medications interact with leukotriene antagonists?

- Aspirin may *increase* the effects of *Accolate®*.

- These medications may *increase* the effect of *Coumadin®* (warfarin); therefore, your doctor may check your blood more often.

- Theophylline may _decrease_ the level of Accolate®.

- Zyflo® may _increase_ the levels of theophylline.

What else should I know about leukotriene antagonists?

• You should continue the use of these agents even if you have a sudden asthma attack.

• Avoid these agents if you have liver disease.

Proper use of aerosol metered dose inhalers (MDIs)

1. Remove the cap on the inhaler. Shake the inhaler very well (at least 60 seconds).

2. Breathe out slowly; blow as much air as you can from your lungs.

3. Hold the inhaler upright and place the mouthpiece two fingerwidths away from your mouth. If this does not work, put the mouthpiece in your mouth and form a tight seal with your lips. Try to keep your tongue out of the way.

4. As you breathe in slowly and deeply, press the inhaler once and continue to breathe in as long as you can. Hold your breath to the count of 10, or as close to that as possible.

5. Breathe out gently. If your doctor has told you to take more than one inhalation of the medication at a time, wait at least one minute, and repeat steps.

6. If you are taking a corticosteroid medication, gargle or rinse your mouth with water after the last puff of each dose.

7. Clean your inhaler at least once a day by removing the cartridge and rinsing the plastic case in warm, running water. Dry the case and replace the cartridge. Store the inhaler in a clean, dry place.

8. You can remove the mouthpiece and place the aerosol canister in a sink of water to see if the MDI is full or empty. If it floats on the top, it is empty and you need a new one. If it sinks to the bottom, it means it is full of medication.

Proper use of dry-powder metered dose inhalers (MDIs)

1. *Flovent*® (fluticasone) Rotadisk: Load the disk into the inhaler before using.

2. *Serevent*® (salmeterol) Diskus: Remove the cap from the inhaler. (The disks are already inside the inhaler.)

3. Breathe out slowly; blow as much air as you can from your lungs.

4. Hold the inhaler upright and place the mouthpiece two fingerwidths away from your mouth.

5. As you breathe in fast and deep, press the inhaler once. (Remember: You must breathe in fast and deep for this type of inhaler.)

6. Hold your breath to the count of 10, or as close to that as possible.

7. Breathe out gently.

* You only need to take one inhalation with the *Serevent*® Diskus. If you are using the *Flovent*® Rotadisk, and your doctor has told you to take more than one inhalation at a time, repeat the steps three times.

Keep these inhalers dry, or the powder will cake. You should use these inhalers within two months of opening the outer foil pouch.

Warning

Leukotriene antagonists may increase the chance of liver problems. Your doctor may check your liver function more often while on these agents. Be sure your doctor knows your full medical history before you use any of these medications.

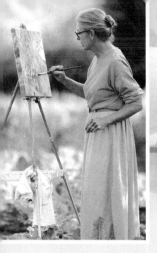

Constipation

What is constipation?

Constipation is the difficulty of passing stools or a decrease in the number of times you have bowel movements. Constipation may cause a feeling of fullness in the stomach or even pain. Older people are five times more likely than younger people to complain of constipation. But most doctors feel that sometimes older people are too worried about having bowel movements every day. There is no "right" number of bowel movements – some people may go twice a day while others may go twice a week. If you're having regular bowel movements and no pain, you're probably not constipated.

The key to managing constipation is prevention. Staying active, drinking plenty of water, and eating plenty of fresh fruits, vegetables, and whole-grain cereals and breads for fiber can help to keep bowel movements regular. Fiber adds bulk to the stool and keeps the bowels moving.

In cases of severe constipation, laxatives – medications that help move the bowels – may be needed for treatment. Laxatives are often needed by people who have constipation as a side effect of medications. Laxatives can cause additional bowel problems, so they should be avoided unless absolutely necessary.

Medications used to treat constipation

Because of the large number of available drug products for the treatment of constipation, a complete listing is not possible. The most commonly used generic names are listed here, as well as some of the more common brand names.

Preventing constipation:

Fiber and Bulk-Forming Agents (BFAs)

Fiber and BFAs help to keep stools soft by increasing the amount of water absorbed in the stomach, making the stools easier to pass. For those who do not get enough fiber in their diets, supplements or BFAs may be a helpful addition. Foods such as whole-grain cereals and vegetables are excellent sources of dietary bulk or fiber. Fiber increases the bulk of stool, keeping the stool soft but well-formed and easier to pass. Raw wheat bran is the oldest and least expensive bulk-forming agent.

Brand Name	Generic
Citrucel®	methylcellulose
Fiberall®	polycarbophil
FiberCon®	polycarbophil
Konsyl®	psyllium
Maltsupex®	malt soup extract
Metamucil®	psyllium
Mitrolan®	polycarbophil
Perdiem® Fiber	psyllium
Unifiber®	cellulose

How do I use bulk-forming laxatives?

Fiber and BFAs must be taken with at least eight ounces of water or juice to prevent stools from becoming hard. If you don't drink enough water or juice, fiber and BFAs may worsen your constipation. The BFAs usually produce a soft, formed stool in one to three days. Remember that any change you make to your diet should be done slowly. Your digestive system may need time to adapt to any changes. Fiber and BFAs may be mixed with food or taken with water shortly after a meal, from one to several times a day.

If you miss a dose, don't be concerned. Take your next scheduled dose as needed. Do not double your dose.

What side effects are possible from the use of bulk-forming laxatives?

More Common

- if too much is taken, may cause diarrhea
- if taken with too little water, may not be effective

Less Common

- stomach bloating and discomfort, especially if taken in large doses; may improve over time
- allergic reactions with products that contain tartrazine used for bronchial asthma. This is more common in patients who are also allergic to aspirin.

Tell your doctor if you have side effects that do not go away over time, are bothersome, or stop you from taking your medication as directed.

What else can bulk-forming laxatives be used for?

Bulk-forming laxatives can also be used for irritable bowel syndrome (a long-term condition that causes diarrhea, constipation, or bowel movements that switch from diarrhea to constipation) or relief of painful bowel movements.

What else should I know about bulk-forming laxatives?

Make sure that you drink at least one additional eight-ounce glass of water with each dose of a BFA.

Stool Softeners

Stool softeners work by holding water in the stool. They may help to reduce the strain or pain of bowel movements.

Brand Name	Generic
Colace®	docusate
Dialose®	docusate
Dialose® Plus	stool softener/stimulant
Peri-Colace®	combinations
Senokot-S®	combinations
Surfak®	docusate

How do I use stool softeners?

Stool softeners should be taken by mouth with at least eight ounces of water or juice once or twice a day. They work best when they are taken before bedtime, so that a soft, formed stool is passed in the morning. Liquid forms that may be taken with milk or juice to improve their flavor are available.

If you miss a dose, don't be concerned. Take your next scheduled dose as needed. Do not double your dose.

What side effects are possible from the use of stool softeners?

- diarrhea
- *increased* absorption of other laxatives

Tell your doctor if you have side effects that do not go away over time, are bothersome, or stop you from taking your medication as directed.

What else should I know about stool softeners?

Occasionally, the stool may become too soft and watery. In this case, reduce the dose.

 ## Warning

Stool-softener/stimulant combinations are not recommended for older people. They have not been shown to work better than when taken separately, and they have a higher rate of complications. Stool softeners can *increase* the amount of stimulant laxatives absorbed into the blood stream, so the combination can produce stronger results and side effects.

Enemas

Enemas work quickly and are very powerful. They work locally in the rectum and the lower large bowel by increasing the amount of fluid there. This stretches the walls of the bowel and causes the feeling of having to do a bowel movement. Enemas may contain plain water or may be combined with additives, such as mineral oil, stimulant agents, or softeners. They should be used only occasionally.

Brand Name	Generic
Fleet's® (various preparations)	enema

How do I use enemas?

Enemas are inserted into the rectum as one single dose.

What side effects are possible from the use of enemas?

More Common

• discomfort and irritation of the rectum

Less Common

• with repeated use: *increase* in diarrhea and water loss which may lead to weakness or shock
• excessive mucus production in the stool

Tell your doctor if you have side effects that do not go away over time, are bothersome, or stop you from taking your medication as directed.

Lubricants

Mineral oil

Mineral oil may be taken alone or in combination with a bulk-forming agent or a mild stimulant laxative. Mineral oil can make moving the bowels easier by lubricating the intestinal tract.

Brand Name	Generic
Agoral®	mineral oil
Kondremul® *Plain*	mineral oil

How do I use lubricants?

Mineral oil is usually taken by mouth, once or twice a day. Mineral oil may also be taken in an enema.

What side effects are possible from the use of lubricants?

- pneumonia if inhaled into the lungs

- liver damage with long-term use

- irritation of the anus and staining of undergarments

Tell your doctor if you have side effects that do not go away over time, are bothersome, or stop you from taking your medication as directed.

Do other medications interact with lubricants?

Mineral oil can decrease the absorption of vitamins and medications.

What else should I know about lubricants?

- Do not lie down after taking mineral oil. This will prevent mineral oil from being inhaled into the lungs.

- Take only as needed. Do not take regularly or problems with vitamin absorption may occur.

Glycerin Suppositories

Glycerin suppositories work by causing the rectum to contract and push out the stool. They also lubricate the anorectal canal and soften stool in the area. Unlike mineral oil, glycerin suppositories do not _decrease_ the absorption of vitamins.

Osmotic Laxatives: Nonabsorbable Salts

Nonabsorbable salts draw fluid into the intestine and increase the contractions that move food through the intestinal tract. Nonabsorbable salts usually work in one to eight hours. They are given when there is a need for rapid relief of constipation. They may also be used to clear the bowel before or after a medical procedure, such as an X-ray. They are very good for treating constipation but should not be used to prevent constipation because their long-term use can cause bowel problems.

Brand Name	Generic
Epsom Salts®	magnesium citrate
Fleet Phospho-Soda®	sodium phosphate
Phillips' Milk of Magnesia®	magnesium oxide

How do I use nonabsorbable salts?

Nonabsorbable salts are often taken by mouth, although enemas are available. Avoid daily use unless prescribed by your doctor.

If you miss a dose, don't be concerned. Take your next scheduled dose as needed. Do not double your dose.

What side effects are possible from the use of nonabsorbable salts?

- excessive gas and cramping (gets better with time)

- watery stools (can lead to dehydration, the loss of too much water from the body)

Tell your doctor if you have side effects that do not go away over time, are bothersome, or stop you from taking your medication as directed.

What else should I know about nonabsorbable salts?

Avoid these laxatives if you have kidney disease. Talk with your doctor before using if you have a history of hypertension (high blood pressure) or congestive heart failure.

 ## Warning

- Nonabsorbable salts may cause life-threatening problems in people with kidney disease.

Osmotic Laxatives: Nonabsorbable Sugars

Lactulose and sorbitol are sugars that cannot be absorbed by the intestine. Like nonabsorbable salts, nonabsorbable sugars draw water into the colon to help make a soft, formed stool. Nonabsorbable sugars are sometimes given to people who have become dependent on other laxatives.

Brand Name	Generic
Chronulac®	lactulose
various	sorbitol

How do I use nonabsorbable sugars?

These agents can be taken once or twice a day with water.

If you miss a dose, don't be concerned. Take your next scheduled dose as needed. Do not double your dose.

What side effects are possible from the use of nonabsorbable sugars?

• a lot of gas and cramping (gets better with time)

• watery stools (can lead to dehydration, the loss of too much water from the body)

Tell your doctor if you have side effects that do not go away over time, are bothersome, or stop you from taking your medication as directed.

Stimulant Laxatives

Stimulant laxatives work by activating the muscles of the bowel. The following are the most commonly used agents:

Brand Name	Generic
Dulcolax®	bisacodyl
Ex-Lax®	senna
Nature's Remedy®	cascara sagrada
Neoloid®	castor oil
Senokot®	senna

Dulcolax® – strong and fast-acting. Oral or suppository form available. Useful for x-ray preparation. May cause irritation of the rectum.

Nature's Remedy® – mild agent that stimulates the large bowel. May cause coloring of intestine with prolonged use. May color the urine.

Neoloid® – too strong for common constipation. May be used for X-ray preparation.

Ex-Lax® – the active ingredient is in many over-the-counter preparations. May cause severe dehydration or rash.

Senokot® – similar to *Nature's Remedy®* but with stronger action. Increases bowel movement and softens the stool.

What else should I know about stimulant laxatives?

Older people should not use stimulant laxatives unless there is an occasional need for rapid relief of constipation. Stimulant laxatives should not be used to prevent constipation except in people using medications that cause constipation, such as narcotics.

Warning

- The stimulant laxatives should not be used daily (for more than a few weeks), unless directed by your doctor.

- Long-term daily use may cause the patient to become dependent (depend on the product for bowel movements all of the time).

Tell your doctor if you have side effects that do not go away over time, are bothersome, or stop you from taking your medication as directed.

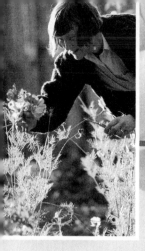

Depression

What is depression?

We all feel a little down or blue sometimes. Many people call these feelings "depression." But, the true medical definition of depression (clinical depression) is more than brief periods of sadness or feeling a little low. Clinical depression is a disorder that can affect the whole body, the way you think and the way you feel.

If you have had four or more of the following symptoms for more than two weeks, you should talk with your doctor because you might have more than the "blues":

- great sadness
- loss of interest in normal activities
- overwhelming hopelessness
- tiredness
- change in appetite (either weight gain or weight loss)
- difficulty concentrating
- problems sleeping
- thoughts of death or suicide
- aches and pains that come back again and again, and are not helped by treatment

Depression is not always noticed in older people. Remember that it is not "normal" for older people to feel depressed. Also, older people may not show the usual symptoms of depression. They may complain of other symptoms, such as headaches, back aches, joint pain, or stomach problems when they are depressed.

Depression seems to be related to abnormal changes in the chemical signals in the brain. Other causes are other illnesses, such as cancer or strokes, certain medications, genetics, personality types, and life events, such as loss of a loved one.

The good news is that depression can often be successfully treated with medication, talking with a trained therapist, or a combination of the two.

Medications used to treat depression

Cyclic Antidepressants

Cyclic antidepressants may take two to six weeks to work. Some of them, such as *Remeron®* (mirtazapine), *Desyrel®* (trazodone) and, especially, *Sinequan®* (doxepin), make you feel drowsy. Others, such as *Norpramin®* (desipramine) and *Pamelor®* (nortriptyline), do not make you feel so drowsy. These may be better at helping older people avoid drowsiness or dizziness during the day.

Of all the antidepressants, *Elavil®* (amitriptyline), *Sinequan®* (doxepin), *Tofranil®* (imipramine) and *Surmontil®* (trimipramine) cause the most side effects in older people and may make them feel the most drowsy. For this reason, these are not recommended for older people.

"▲" Indicates medications that are <u>generally not recommended</u> for use in older people. Do not stop taking these medications unless directed

Brand Name	Generic
▲ *Elavil®*	amitriptyline
▲ *Sinequan®*	doxepin
▲ *Surmontil®*	trimipramine
▲ *Tofranil®*	imipramine
Asendin®	amoxapine
Desyrel®	trazodone
Ludiomil®	maprotiline
Norpramin®	desipramine
Pamelor®	nortriptyline
Remeron®	mirtazapine
Vivactil®	protriptyline

by your doctor. They may be required under special circumstances. Talk to your doctor to see if this medication is right for you.

How do I use cyclic antidepressants?

These medications are usually taken by mouth, once a day at bedtime. Antidepressants take time to work. You should never stop taking these before talking with your doctor. Your doctor may start with a low dose, increasing it slowly until the right dose is reached.

If you miss a dose of this medication, take it as soon as possible. However, if it is almost time for your next dose, skip the missed dose and go back to the dosing schedule. Do not double your dose. It is very important to take your medication exactly as directed by your doctor. NEVER stop taking your prescription medications without talking with your doctor.

What side effects are possible from the use of cyclic antidepressants?

More Common
- dry mouth
- sleepiness
- constipation
- light-headedness upon standing
- blurred vision
- increased or decreased interest in sex
- painful ejaculation or impotence

Less Common
- confusion
- allergic skin reactions
- difficulty urinating
- blurred vision and worsening of glaucoma (an eye disease)
- rapid heartbeat
- weight gain

Rare
- seizures
- abnormal heart rhythms

Tell your doctor if you have side effects that do not go away over time, are bothersome, or stop you from taking your medication as directed.

Do other medications interact with cyclic antidepressants?

- Use of cyclic antidepressants and clonidine together may raise blood pressure to dangerous levels.

- *Thorazine*® (chlorpromazine), *Mellaril*® (thioridazine), *Stelazine*® (trifluoperazine), *Navane*® (thiothixene), and *Prolixin*® (fluphenazine) may _increase_ the effects of cyclic antidepressants.

- Antihistamines and anticholinergic medications used in Parkinson's disease may _increase_ the side effects of cyclic antidepressants.

What else can cyclic antidepressants be used for?

Cyclic antidepressants can also be used for long-term pain, phobias (abnormal fears), urinary incontinence (inability to control flow of urine), and eating disorders.

What else should I know about cyclic antidepressants?

- These medications may worsen constipation, urinary retention (difficulty urinating), or changes in blood pressure upon standing up from a sitting or lying position.

- People with glaucoma (an eye disease), heart disease, liver failure, a history of seizures, or benign prostatic hyperplasia should not use certain _tricyclic_ antidepressants without checking with their doctors.

 # Warning

- Since these medications may make you unsteady on your feet, you may be at risk for a fall which can lead to a broken bone. If you have a history of falling, be sure to tell your doctor. Your doctor may be able to change your medication to reduce your risk of falling.

- MAOIs (monoamine oxidase inhibitors) must be stopped two weeks before starting any cyclic antidepressant.

- Cyclic antidepressants should be stopped two weeks before starting on MAOIs. (The time off between antidepressants depends on the type of medication. Check with your doctor or pharmacist before starting a new antidepressant.)

- Patients who have been taking this medication for more than one month should lower the dose gradually when stopping the medication. Abruptly stopping this medication could cause withdrawal symptoms.

Ritalin® (Methylphenidate)

Brand Name	Generic
Ritalin®	methylphenidate

Ritalin® is a stimulant. It can help relieve depression in older people who are withdrawn, drowsy, slow-moving, and sleepy. It is particularly helpful in depressed people who stop eating. Unlike other medications to treat depression, this medication can produce improvement within a day or two.

How do I use Ritalin®?

Ritalin® is taken by mouth, usually two times a day with breakfast and lunch to avoid insomnia (trouble sleeping).

If you miss a dose of this medication, take it as soon as possible. However, if it is almost time for your next dose, skip the missed dose and go back to the dosing schedule. Do not double your dose. It is very important to take your medication exactly as directed by your doctor. NEVER stop taking your prescription medications without talking with your doctor.

What side effects are possible from the use of Ritalin®?

More Common
- mild increase in blood pressure
- increased heartbeat
- increased appetite
- insomnia

Less Common
- severe high blood pressure
- agitation (a "hyper" feeling) and anxiety
- chest pain (angina)

Tell your doctor if you have side effects that do not go away over time, are bothersome, or stop you from taking your medication as directed.

What else should I know about Ritalin®?

- Use caution if you are currently taking anti-arrhythmics due to the potential increase of your heartbeat.

- This medication is usually for short-term use until other antidepressants begin to work.

- If you have been taking this medication for more than one month, talk to your doctor to see if you still need it. Do not stop taking this unless told to by your doctor.

Selective Serotonin Re-Uptake Inhibitors (SSRIs)

These are relatively new medications.

Brand Name	Generic
Paxil®	paroxetine
Prozac®	fluoxetine
Zoloft®	sertraline

How do I use selective serotonin re-uptake inhibitors (SSRIs)?

These medications are taken by mouth once a day, usually in the morning, with or without food. These medications tend to cause a loss of appetite. SSRIs take time to work (two to four weeks). Your doctor may start with a low dose, increasing it slowly to reach a level that works for you.

If you miss a dose, don't be concerned. Take your next scheduled dose as needed. Do not double your dose. It is very important to take your medication exactly as directed by your doctor. NEVER stop taking your prescription medications without talking with your doctor.

What side effects are possible with SSRIs?

More Common
• headache
• anxiety
• nervousness
• dizziness

- loss of appetite
- nausea
- diarrhea
- drowsiness
- insomnia (trouble sleeping)
- decreased interest in sex
- abnormal ejaculation
- tremor (shakiness)

Less Common
- constipation
- stomach pain
- rash

Tell your doctor if you have side effects that do not go away over time, are bothersome, or stop you from taking your medication as directed.

Do other medications interact with SSRIs?

The following medications may increase SSRI side effects:

- other antidepressants
- *Haldol®* (haloperidol)
- *Lithonate®* (lithium)
- *Lithotabs®* (lithium)
- *Tagamet®* (cimetidine)
- *Valium®* (diazepam)

SSRIs may increase the action of *Coumadin®* (warfarin). Be sure to tell your doctor all of the medications you are taking.

What else can SSRIs be used for?

Obsessive-Compulsive Disorder.

What else should I know about SSRIs?

People with kidney or liver disease should use SSRIs with caution.

 ## Warning

- Do not mix monoamine oxidase inhibitors (MAOIs) with any antidepressant agents.

- MAOIs must be stopped two weeks before starting any other SSRI antidepressant.

- Other antidepressants should be stopped two to six weeks before starting on MAOIs. (The time off between antidepressants depends on the type of medication.)

- Patients who have been taking this medication for more than one month should lower the dose gradually when stopping the medication. Abruptly stopping this medication could cause withdrawal symptoms.

Effexor® (Venlafaxine)

Effexor® is a new agent to treat depression. As with most antidepressants, you may need to take *Effexor®* for several weeks before you see an improvement.

Brand Name	Generic
Effexor®	venlafaxine

How do I use Effexor®?

Effexor® is taken by mouth two or three times a day, with food. Your doctor may start with a low dose, increasing it slowly until the right dose is found for you.

If you miss a dose of this medication, take it as soon as possible. However, if it is almost time for your next dose, skip the missed dose and go back to the dosing schedule. Do not double your dose. It is very important to take your medication exactly as directed by your doctor. NEVER stop taking your prescription medications without talking with your doctor.

What side effects are possible from the use of Effexor®?

More Common
- headache
- nervousness
- dizziness
- long-lasting drowsiness
- visual changes
- nausea
- insomnia (trouble sleeping)
- dry mouth

Less Common
- fast heartbeat
- problems urinating
- ringing in ears
- rash

Tell your doctor if you have side effects that do not go away over time, are bothersome, or stop you from taking your medication as directed.

Do other medications interact with Effexor®?

- *Tagamet®* (cimetidine) may increase the effects of *Effexor®*.

- Be careful when using alcohol (beer, wine, liquor, etc.) and other medications that may make you drowsy.

What else should I know about Effexor®?

- People with heart, kidney, or liver disease should use *Effexor®* with caution.

- *Effexor®* increases blood pressure; therefore, people with poorly controlled hypertension (high blood pressure) should avoid this medication.

 ## Warning

- Do not mix monoamine oxidase inhibitors (MAOIs) with any other antidepressant.

- MAOIs must be stopped two weeks before starting any other antidepressant.

- Other antidepressants should be stopped two to six weeks before starting on MAOIs. (The time off between antidepressants depends on the type of medication).

- Patients who have been taking this medication for more than two weeks should slowly lower the dose before stopping the medication. Stopping this medication abruptly may cause withdrawal symptoms.

Serzone® (Nefazodone)

Serzone® is a new agent to treat depression. Like most antidepressants, you may need to take *Serzone®* for several weeks before you see an improvement.

Brand Name	Generic
Serzone®	nefazodone

How do I use Serzone®?

Serzone® is usually taken two times a day. You may take this medication with food if you experience an upset stomach. As stated above, Serzone® will need time to take effect. Your doctor may start with a low dose, increasing it slowly until the right dose is found for you.

If you miss a dose of this medication, take it as soon as possible. However, if it is almost time for your next doses, skip the missed dose and go back to the dosing schedule. Do not double your dose. It is very important to take your medication exactly as directed by your doctor. NEVER stop taking your prescription medications without talking with your doctor.

What side effects are possible from the use of Serzone®?

More Common

- headache
- insomnia (trouble sleeping)
- agitation ("hyper" feeling)
- drowsiness
- nausea
- dizziness
- dry mouth

Less Common

- dizziness upon standing
- constipation
- problems urinating

Rare

- lasting, painful erection (priaprism)

Tell your doctor if you have side effects that do not go away over time, are bothersome, or stop you from taking your medication as directed.

Do other medications interact with Serzone®?

- You should not take the non-sedating antihistamines *Seldane*® (terfena-dine) or *Hismanal*® (astemizole) with *Serzone*® due to possible life-threatening heart problems.

- Serzone may increase the effect of *Xanax*® (alprazolam) and *Halcion*® (triazolam).

 Warning

- Do not mix monoamine oxidase inhibitors (MAOIs) with any other antidepressants.

- MAOIs must be stopped two weeks before starting any other antide-pressant.

- Other antidepressants should be stopped two to six weeks before starting on MAOIs (The time off between antidepressants depends on the type of drug).

- Patients who have been taking this medication for more than one month should lower the dose gradually when stopping the medication. Abruptly stopping this medication could cause withdrawal symptoms.

What else should I know about Serzone®?

- People with heart, kidney, or liver disease should use this medication with caution.

- Call your doctor immediately if you have a lasting, painful erection.

Wellbutrin® (Bupropion)

Wellbutrin® may be effective when other agents have not been effective. As with other antidepressants, it may take several weeks to see improvements in your mood.

How do I use Wellbutrin®?

Wellbutrin® should be taken by mouth two or three times a day. You should never stop taking this medication before talking with your doctor. Your doctor may start with a low dose, increasing it slowly to find the right dose for you.

If you miss a dose of this medication, take it as soon as possible. However, if it is almost time for your next dose, skip the missed dose and go back to the dosing schedule. Do not double your dose. It is very important to take your medication exactly as directed by your doctor. NEVER stop taking your prescription medications without talking with your doctor.

What side effects are possible from the use of Wellbutrin®?

More Common
- constipation
- dry mouth
- decreased appetite
- dizziness
- nausea
- tremors

Less Common
- blurry vision
- trouble sleeping
- drowsiness

Tell your doctor if you have side effects that do not go away over time, are bothersome, or stop you from taking your medication as directed.

Do other medications interact with Wellbutrin®?

• The effects of seizure medications may be _decreased_ when taken with _Wellbutrin®_.

• The effects of _Sinemet®_ (levodopa) and _Nardil®_ (phenelzine) and _Parnate®_ (tranylcypromine) (both are brand names of MAOIs) may be _increased_ when taken with _Wellbutrin®_.

What else should I know about Wellbutrin®?

Wellbutrin® may _increase_ the chance for seizures. It should be used cautiously if you have a history of seizures or are on anticonvulsants.

 ## Warning

• Do not mix monoamine oxidase inhibitors (MAOIs) with any other antidepressant.

• MAOIs must be stopped two weeks before starting any other antidepressant.

• Other antidepressants should be stopped two to six weeks before starting on MAOIs. (The time off between antidepressants depends on the type of medication.)

Monoamine Oxidase Inhibitors (MAOIs)

These antidepressants are different from the cyclic antidepressants. They have their own side effects and precautions. Most often, they are given if cyclic antidepressants have not worked or cannot be used for other reasons.

Brand Name	Generic
Nardil®	phenelzine
Parnate®	tranylcypromine

How do I use monoamine oxidase inhibitors (MAOIs)?

MAOIs are taken two or three times daily. People who take MAOIs must follow a strict diet (see below). MAOIs should be taken apart from meals and other medications.

As with other antidepressants, MAOIs take time to work. Your doctor may start with a low dose, increasing it slowly to find the dose that works for you.

If you miss a dose of this medication, take it as soon as possible. However, if it is almost time for your next dose, skip the missed dose and go back to the dosing schedule. Do not double your dose. It is very important to take your medication exactly as directed by your doctor. NEVER stop taking your prescription medications without talking with your doctor.

What side effects are possible from the use of MAOIs?

More Common

- light-headedness upon standing

Less Common

- drowsiness
- constipation
- dry mouth
- blurred vision
- weight gain

Rare

- impotence
- low white blood cell count
- sensitivity to light
- insomnia (trouble sleeping)
- skin rash
- tremors (shakiness)
- severe high blood pressure
- water retention

Tell your doctor if you have side effects that do not go away over time, are bothersome, or stop you from taking your medication as directed.

Do other medications interact with MAOIs?

The following should be avoided as they may cause extremely high blood pressure, even death:

- Some foods to avoid: tyramine-containing foods and beverages, including aged cheese, red wine, kippered or pickled herring, chicken livers, figs, fava beans, chocolate, and beer.

- Some medications to avoid: amphetamines, decongestants that are frequently found in cold or asthma preparations, *Sinemet*® (levodopa), *Aldomet*® (methyldopa), *Ritalin*® (methylphenidate), *Demerol*® (meperidine) and other antidepressants.

What else should I know about monoamine oxidase inhibitors (MAOIs)?

- Follow the recommended diet exactly as described while on the medication and for three weeks after stopping the MAOI.

- Talk with your physician or pharmacist before starting any new medications or eating unusual foods.

- Wear a MedicAlert bracelet.

• See a physician immediately if you develop headache, abnormal heartbeat, nausea, vomiting, or sweating.

 # Warning

• MAOIs interact with certain foods and many other medications, leading to serious, even life-threatening side effects. For example, the combination of MAOIs with certain foods can cause sudden and severe elevations in blood pressure. Ask your physician for a complete list of foods and medications to avoid when taking MAOIs.

• MAOIs should not be taken by people who drink more than three alcoholic drinks (beer, wine, whiskey, etc.) per day or suffer from severe heart, liver, or kidney disease, or from poorly controlled high blood pressure.

• MAOIs must be stopped two weeks before starting any other antidepressant.

• Other antidepressants should be stopped two to six weeks before starting on MAOIs. (The time off between antidepressants depends on the type of medication.) Check with your doctor or pharmacist before starting a new antidepressant.

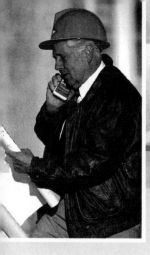

Diabetes

What is diabetes?

Diabetes is a disease that affects the way the body is able to handle food and sugar. Diabetes is caused by not having enough insulin or insulin that does not function as well as it should. This leads to high blood sugar (glucose).

After eating a snack or a meal, your body changes your food into a special type of sugar called glucose. Glucose is a type of fuel that your body uses.

The pancreas is an organ that helps to control the amount of glucose in the body. The pancreas makes insulin, a protein, to help break down glucose. People with diabetes do not have enough insulin, or their bodies cannot use the insulin in the right way.

Symptoms of diabetes may include feeling tired, feeling more thirsty, and needing to urinate more often. Other symptoms include increased appetite, slow wound-healing, blurred vision, tingling in the hands or feet, and weight loss. Some older people with diabetes do not have any symptoms or only very mild symptoms, others may have very severe symptoms, even coma. Also, some older people mistake these symptoms for normal signs of aging.

If left untreated, over the long term, diabetes can cause blindness, nerve damage, need for amputations, and kidney failure. Diabetes may also increase your risk of heart disease and stroke. Controlling diabetes may lessen the chance of these problems developing. Diabetes may be controlled by a combination of a special diet, regular exercise, and medication.

Special instructions for all patients with diabetes

- If you have diabetes, talk with your doctor before starting a new exercise plan or making any changes in your diet. Changes in your diet and exercise can affect the amount of medication you need to control your blood sugar.

- Always wear a MedicAlert bracelet to let your healthcare providers know you have diabetes. You can get these at most pharmacies.

- Never skip meals or any medication doses unless directed to do so by your doctor.

- Blood sugar monitoring at home is a good way to keep watch on diabetes. Blood sugar monitoring will show you how well your blood sugar is controlled and show the effects of any changes in your diet, exercise, or insulin dosages. If you have a home blood glucose monitor, use it as directed by your doctor. Be sure to take the results to your doctor, so your medication and treatment plan can be changed if necessary. People who monitor their glucose at home have more control over their disease and often have fewer symptoms. If you do not have a monitor, talk with your doctor to see if one would be right for you.

- All diabetics are at risk for foot sores. Ask your doctor about how you should check your feet daily. Have regular foot exams to reduce your risk of infection, resulting in amputation (surgery to remove all or part of the foot).

Warning for all diabetic medication

- Low blood sugar (hypoglycemia) can occur if your body has too much insulin or too much diabetes medicine. If low blood sugar is not corrected, it can cause severe illness, even coma.

- Missing or delaying a meal can cause hypoglycemia.

- More physical activity than usual, like housecleaning, yard work or going to the market, can cause low blood sugar.

The symptoms of low blood sugar are:

- weakness, tiredness
- nervousness, feeling excited
- confusion
- double vision
- sweating
- dizziness
- heart palpitations or increased heartbeat
- rapid, shallow breathing
- hunger
- unconsciousness
- nausea
- pale, moist skin

Most low blood sugar effects may be corrected by eating or drinking sugar (usually a glass of fruit juice or several pieces of candy), but sugar must be eaten as soon as possible to avoid more serious problems. If you have a home glucose monitor and develop these symptoms, check your blood sugar to see if you have low blood sugar. Make sure your family and close friends also know how to recognize and manage these problems. Always carry some form of sugar with you. You may want to ask your doctor or pharmacist about glucose tablets.

Alcohol (beer, wine, whiskey, etc.) should not be used or used only in small amounts. In large amounts it can cause low blood sugar. Alcohol can also prevent you from noticing that you have low blood sugar.

Beta-blockers, such as *Inderal*® (propranolol), *Tenormin*® (atenolol), *Lopressor*® (metoprolol), etc., may block the signs of low blood sugar in your body like increased heartbeat. It can be dangerous if you have low blood sugar and do not know it. If you take beta-blockers, check your blood sugar as directed.

Medications used to treat diabetes

Oral Hypoglycemics (Blood Sugar Pills)

Oral hypoglycemics cause the pancreas to release insulin and increase the effects of insulin on the body. Insulins and oral hypoglycemics work for different amounts of time in the body.

"▲" Indicates medications that are <u>generally not recommended</u> for use in older people. Do not stop taking these medications unless directed by your doctor. They may be required under special circumstances. Talk to your doctor to see if this medication is right for you. (See "Warning for all diabetic medication" on page 83.)

Brand Name	Generic
▲ *Diabinese®*	chlorpropamide
Amaryl®	glimepiride
DiaBeta®	glyburide
Dymelor®	acetohexamide
Glucotrol®	glipizide
Glynase®	glyburide
Micronase®	glyburide
Orinase®	tolbutamide
Tolinase®	tolazamide

How do I use oral hypoglycemics?

Oral hypoglycemics are taken either once a day before breakfast or in divided doses before meals.

If you miss a dose of this medication, take it as soon as possible. However, if it is almost time for your next dose, skip the missed dose and go back to the dosing schedule. Do not double your dose. It is very important to take your medication exactly as directed by your doctor. NEVER stop taking your prescription medications without talking with your doctor.

What side effects are possible from the use of hypoglycemics?

More Common

- diarrhea
- upset stomach
- nausea
- skin redness or flushing from drinking alcohol (beer, wine, whiskey, etc.)
- sun sensitivity (use sunscreen and protective clothing or avoid sun exposure)

Less Common

- allergic skin reactions – rashes that usually go away without treatment (report any such reactions to your doctor)
- immune system problems
- lingering sore throats, persistent infections, bleeding, bruising, or change in the color of stool, urine, or skin (report such symptoms or signs to your doctor)

Tell your doctor if you have side effects that do not go away over time, are bothersome, or stop you from taking your medication as directed.

Do other medications interact with hypoglycemics?

The following medications may _decrease_ the effect of oral hypoglycemics and *result in an _increase_ in blood sugar levels (hyperglycemia):*

- corticosteroids (such as prednisone)
- *Dilantin*® (phenytoin)
- thiazide diuretics (such as hydrochlorathiazide)
- thyroid medications

- *Questran*® (cholestyramine)
- *Rifadin*® (rifampin)

The following medications may _increase_ the effect of the oral hypoglycemics and *result in a _decrease_ in blood sugar levels (hypoglycemia)*:

- chloramphenicol
- *Atromid-S*® (clofibrate)
- *Diflucan*® (fluconazole)
- *Lopid*® (gemfibrozil)
- *Parnate*® (phenelzine), *Nardil*® (tranylcypromine)
- *Butazolidin*® (phenylbutazone)
- aspirin
- *Anturane*® (sulfinpyrazone)
- *Septra*®, *Bactrim*® (trimethoprim/sulfamethoxazole)
- *Coumadin*® (warfarin)

Oral hypoglycemics can _increase_ the effects of blood thinners, such as *Coumadin*®, and _increase_ bleeding.

Warning

- The longer-acting agent *Diabinese*® (chlorpropamide) generally should not be used by older people with diabetes. It can cause many side effects, especially long-term low blood sugar. Shorter-acting agents are much safer for most older people. *Diabinese*® may reduce the amount of fluid removed from the body by the kidneys. If too much fluid stays in the body, it can cause swelling of the hands, face, or ankles. This medication can also lead to problems with the salt levels in the blood. If you are taking *Diabinese*®, talk with your doctor to see if it is the right medication for you. But never stop taking the medication without speaking to your doctor.

- With longer-acting agents, low blood sugar may continue for some time. If symptoms do not reverse quickly by taking some sugar, seek medical attention quickly. If you are taking oral medication, especially one like *Diabinese*®, you will have to be extra careful. Your symptoms may return hours after you have taken sugar. You will have to watch your blood sugar and your symptoms closely for several days after having low blood sugar.

- See "Warning for all diabetic medication" on page 83.

Oral Antiglycemics

These medications lower blood sugar closer to normal. They cannot cause low blood sugar or blood sugar below normal (hypoglycemia) unless they are given with insulin or oral hypoglycemics.

Brand Name	Generic
Glucophage®	metformin
Precose®	acarbose
Rezulin®	troglitazone

Precose® (Acarbose)

How do I use Precose®?

Take Precose® three times a day at the very beginning of each main meal (just before your first bite).

If you miss a dose, don't be concerned. Take your next scheduled dose with your next meal. Do not double your dose. It is very important to take your medication exactly as directed by your doctor. NEVER stop taking your prescription medications without talking with your doctor.

What side effects are possible from the use of Precose®?

- stomach pain, diarrhea, gas (these often decrease over time)
- increased liver enzymes
- low calcium and vitamin B_6 levels

Tell your doctor if you have side effects that do not go away over time, are bothersome, or stop you from taking your medication as directed.

Do other medications interact with Precose®?

- *Lanoxin®* (digoxin) absorption into the bloodstream may be <u>decreased</u> by *Precose®*.

- *Precose®* effectiveness may be <u>decreased</u> when taken with digestive enzyme medications such as *Creon 10®*, *Pancrease®*, *Viokase®* (pancrelipase).

 # Warning

- Acarbose may cause low blood sugar (hypoglycemia) when given with insulin or oral hypoglycemic medications. (See "Warning for all diabetic medication" on page 83.)

- If you develop low blood sugar while taking *Precose®*, regular table sugar will *NOT* work to raise your blood sugar to a safe level. You will need to have a special glucose preparation to raise your blood sugar.

- Ask your doctor or pharmacist to make sure you have the right glucose preparation on hand in case it is needed.

Glucophage® (Metformin)

How do I use Glucophage®?

Glucophage® is taken twice daily – once with your breakfast and once with your evening meal. If you are prescribed the medication three times daily, take it with your breakfast, lunch, and dinner.

If you miss a dose of this medication, take it as soon as possible. However, if it is almost time for your next dose, skip the missed dose and go back to the dosing schedule. Do not double your dose. It is very important to take your medication exactly as directed by your doctor. NEVER stop taking your prescription medications without talking with your doctor.

What side effects are possible from the use of Glucophage®?

More Common

- diarrhea
- nausea
- vomiting
- bloating (usually when treatment is started)
- low vitamin B_{12} blood levels

Rare/Severe

Lactic acidosis (a build-up of acid in the body) is rare, but sometimes fatal. Call your doctor immediately if you develop these symptoms:

- muscle pain
- extreme tiredness
- severe stomach discomfort
- difficulty breathing
- nausea

Tell your doctor if you have side effects that do not go away over time, are bothersome, or stop you from taking your medication as directed.

Do other medications interact with Glucophage®?

- If you are taking *Glucophage*® with oral hypoglycemics or insulin, you can get low blood sugar. (See "Warnings for all diabetic medication" on page 83.)

- *Tagamet*® (cimetidine) can increase the effects of *Glucophage*®. Do not take OTC medications before talking to your doctor or pharmacist.

- *Lasix*® (furosemide) and *Procardia*® (nifedipine) can increase effects of *Glucophage*®.

 # Warning

- *Glucophage*® cannot be used by patients who have kidney disease. Tell your doctor if you have kidney problems.

- *Glucophage*® may cause hypoglycemia when given with insulin or oral hypoglycemic medications. (See "Warning for all diabetic medication" on page 83.)

- *Glucophage*® should be stopped 48 hours before you have surgery and before some special laboratory tests that involve contrast dye. Ask your doctor about this if you have any upcoming procedures.

- Do not drink alcohol (beer, wine, whiskey, etc.) while taking *Glucophage*®. It increases your chance of developing lactic acidosis, which can cause death.

Rezulin® (Troglitazone)

How do I use Rezulin®?

Rezulin® is usually taken once a day with a meal.

If you miss a dose of this medication, take it as soon as possible. However, if it is almost time for your next dose, skip the missed dose and go back to the dosing schedule. Do not double your dose. It is very important to take your medication exactly as directed by your doctor. NEVER stop taking your prescription medications without talking with your doctor.

What side effects are possible from the use of Rezulin®?

Common
• jaundice (yellowing of the skin)
• hepatitis

Rare
• liver failure – symptoms include nausea, vomiting, stomach pain, tiredness, dark urine or jaundice (yellowing of the skin and whites of the eyes)

Tell your doctor if you have side effects that do not go away over time, are bothersome, or stop you from taking your medication as directed.

Do other medications interact with Rezulin®?

• *Questran®* (cholestyramine) <u>decreases</u> the effectiveness of *Rezulin®*. These two medications should not be taken together. If you are taking *Questran®*, talk with your doctor.

• *Rezulin®* <u>decreases</u> the effect of *Seldane®* (terfenadine).

 # Warning

• In rare cases, *Rezulin®* can cause liver failure. Alert your doctor immediately if you develop nausea, vomiting, stomach pain, tiredness, dark urine or jaundice (yellowing of the skin and the whites of the eyes).

• *Rezulin®* may cause low blood sugar when given with insulin or oral hypoglycemic medications. (See "Warning for all diabetic medication" on page 83.)

Insulin

When diet, exercise, weight reduction, and oral medications do not control blood sugar, the older person with diabetes may require insulin. People who do not normally require insulin may need to take it during times of severe stress, such as during a major illness or following surgery.

How do I use insulin?

Insulins are grouped according to how quickly they begin to work and how long they stay in the body. Short-acting insulin (regular) goes to work quickly but works for a shorter period of time; long-acting insulin (NPH and Lente) stays in the body longer. People with diabetes may take a combination of short-, intermediate-, and long-acting insulins once or several times a day.

Insulin is injected just under the skin into the thigh, stomach, or upper arm. Rotating the sites in the same area from day to day will prevent damage to the tissue. There are several new instruments that can help you measure and inject your insulin (magnifiers, insulin pens, cartridges, etc.) Ask your doctor or pharmacist for advice about these instruments.

If you miss a dose of this medication, take it as soon as possible. However, if it is almost time for your next dose, skip the missed dose and go back to the dosing schedule. Do not double your dose. It is very important to take your medication exactly as directed by your doctor. NEVER stop taking your prescription medications without talking with your doctor.

What side effects are possible from the use of insulin?

- Hypoglycemia (low blood sugar) – See "Warning for all diabetic medication" on page 83.

- Lipodystrophies – either lumps of fat or a loss of tissue under the skin, which can occur at the injection site. They cause dimpling of the skin in the area and occur after repeated injections in one place. Rotating injection sites helps prevent this problem.

- Problems with vision – the lens of the eye responds to any rapid change in blood sugar. When you start insulin (or if your blood sugar is not well controlled), your vision may become blurry. This vision problem comes and goes and is different from the very serious eye problems that may occur after years of diabetes.

Tell your doctor if you have side effects that do not go away over time, are bothersome, or stop you from taking your medication as directed.

Do other medications interact with insulin?

The following medications may <u>decrease</u> the hypoglycemic (sugar lowering) effect of insulin and cause high blood sugar:

- AIDS antiviral medications
- *Cardizem*® (diltiazem)
- corticosteroids
- *Diamox*® (acetazolamide)
- *Dilantin*® (phenytoin)
- diuretics (water pills)
- *Eskalith*® (lithium)
- isoniazid
- *Miacalcin*® (calcitonin)
- morphine
- niacin
- *Premarin*®, *Ogen*® (estrogens)
- *Thorazine*®, *Stelazine*® (phenothiazines)
- thyroid medications

The following medications may <u>increase</u> the hypoglycemic (sugar lowering) effect of insulin and cause low blood sugar:

- ACE inhibitors
- alcohol (beer, wine, whiskey, etc.)
- *Anturane*® (sulfinpyrazone)
- aspirin
- *Atromid-S*® (clofibrate)
- *Butazolidin*® (phenylbutazone)
- *Ismelin*® (guanethidine)

- *Parnate*® (phenelzine)(MAO inhibitors)
- *Nardil*® (tranylcypromine)
- *Pentam*®, *NebuPent*® (pentamidine)
- *Septra*®, *Bactrim*® (trimethoprim/sulfamethoxazole)
- tetracycline antibiotics

What else should I know about insulin?

If it is necessary to rotate injection sites, this should be done around one area of the body. Changing injection sites too drastically may change the amount of insulin that is absorbed into your body.

Warning

- Never change the kind of insulin you use or your dose unless told to by your doctor.

- Kidney or liver disease may increase the effects of human insulin. Tell your doctor if you have kidney or liver problems.

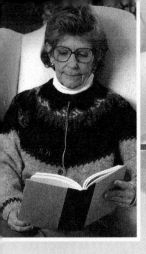

Glaucoma

What is glaucoma?

Glaucoma is a disease that affects the eyes. Glaucoma occurs when there is too much fluid pressure in the eye, which causes damage. If glaucoma is not treated, it can result in a slow loss of vision.

If glaucoma is discovered early and treated, it can usually be controlled. Glaucoma rarely causes any symptoms in its early stages. It is important to get regular eye exams that test your vision and eye muscles, and check for glaucoma, every two to three years. If your family has a history of eye disease or if you have diabetes, you may need eye exams more often.

Glaucoma may be treated by eye drops, eye ointments, oral medication, laser treatments, or surgery.

Medications used to treat glaucoma

The medications used to treat glaucoma are usually eye drops, gels, or ointments. These agents work locally in the eye. Small amounts of medication are absorbed into the blood stream. The low absorption in the bloodstream reduces drug interactions and side effects. However, they may still occur.

Miotics

Miotic agents lower the pressure of the fluid in the eye. The short-acting miotics, such as pilocarpine, are generally good medications for treatment of glaucoma. Miotic agents generally have few side effects. People with unremoved cataracts may find that miotics worsen vision.

Short-acting:

Brand Name	Generic
Adsorbocarpine®	pilocarpine
Isopto® Carbachol	carbachol
Isopto® Carpine	pilocarpine
Pilocar®	pilocarpine
P.V. Carpine®	pilocarpine

Long-acting:

Brand Name	Generic
Floropryl®	isoflurophate
Humorsol®	demecarium
Phospholine Iodide®	echothiophate

How do I use miotics?

These medications are used as eye drops two to four times a day. Newer gel preparations are put into the eye at night. There are also specialized delivery systems that are placed under the eyelid and left in for up to a week. See directions for eye drops and ointments on pages 108–109.

If you miss a dose of this medication, take it as soon as possible. However, if it is almost time for your next dose, skip the missed dose and go back to the dosing schedule. Do not double your dose. It is very important to take your medication exactly as directed by your doctor. NEVER stop taking your prescription medications without talking with your doctor.

What side effects are possible from the use of miotics?

More Common

- miosis, or narrowing of the pupil of the eye (this may be a particular problem for people with cataracts)
- blurred vision or changes in near or far vision
- poor night vision due to pupil narrowing
- burning and irritation (usually an initial reaction)

Less Common

- headache
- twitching of the eyelids
- eye pain
- nasal congestion and tearing
- conjunctivitis (redness and irritation of the eye)

Rare

- increased sweating
- mouth watering
- nausea
- diarrhea
- tremors (shakiness)
- vomiting
- wheezing

Tell your doctor if you have side effects that do not go away over time, are bothersome, or stop you from taking your medication as directed.

What else should I know about miotics?

- Miotic agents reduce vision in dim light; therefore, driving at night may be dangerous.

- When starting or stopping miotic agents, a change in the prescription for your glasses or contact lenses may be needed.

- Use the eye gel preparations in the same way as eye ointments.

Epinephrine and Epinephrine-Like Agents

Epinephrine reduces pressure caused by the fluid in the eye. It is especially useful for people who cannot tolerate the miotics and for older people with cataracts.

Brand Name	Generic
Alphagan®	brimonidine
Epifrin®	epinephrine
Glaucon®	epinephrine
Propine®	dipivefrin

How do I use epinephrine and epinephrine-like agents?

Epinephrine eye drops are generally used once or twice a day. See directions on page 108 for how to use your eye drops.

These medications may be used at any time without concern about meals or other medications, unless your doctor gives you special directions.

Epinephrine is also available in combination with pilocarpine. It is usually given one to four times a day. When it is used four times a day, more epinephrine may be given than is necessary. As with many other medications, it may be better to use each agent separately.

If you miss a dose of this medication, take it as soon as possible. However, if it is almost time for your next dose, skip the missed dose and go back to the dosing schedule. Do not double your dose. It is very important to take your medication exactly as directed by your doctor. NEVER stop taking your prescription medications without talking with your doctor.

What side effects are possible from the use of epinephrine and epinephrine-like agents?

More Common

- wide pupils (blurred vision)
- headache or brow ache
- stinging, burning, eye irritation
- watery eyes

Less Common

- eye pain
- sweating
- increased blood pressure
- pallor (pale skin)
- trembling (shakiness)
- staining of soft contact lenses
- fast or irregular heartbeat

Tell your doctor if you have side effects that do not go away over time, are bothersome, or stop you from taking your medication as directed.

What else should I know about epinephrine and epinephrine-like agents?

• These agents should be kept away from heat and light, which break the medicine down. If the liquid turns brown, throw away immediately. Do not use it.

• You should remove your contact lenses before using *Alphagan®* (brimonidine), and wait at least 15 minutes after using the drops before replacing contact lenses.

 ## Warning

If you have a history of heartbeat irregularities, high blood pressure, overactive thyroid, recent heart attack, or heart disease, be sure to tell your eye doctor.

Topical Beta-Blockers

These medications reduce pressure in the eye by blocking fluid from being formed. They are excellent choices to use instead of pilocarpine, especially in older patients with cataracts. They are also a good choice when epinephrine is not effective or cannot be tolerated.

Brand Name	Generic
Betagan®	levobunolol
Betoptic®	betaxolol
Ocupress®	carteolol
OptiPranolol®	metipranolol
Timoptic®	timolol
Timoptic-XE®	timolol

How do I use topical beta-blockers?

Beta-blockers are applied as eye drops and are generally used once or twice a day. They may be taken without concern about meals or other medications. See page 108 for directions on how to use eye drops.

If you miss a dose of this medication, take it as soon as possible. However, if it is almost time for your next dose, skip the missed dose and go back to the dosing schedule. Do not double your dose. It is very important to take your medication exactly as directed by your doctor. NEVER stop taking your prescription medications without talking with your doctor.

What side effects are possible from the use of topical beta-blockers?

More Common

- eye irritation with redness and swelling
- blurred vision

Less Common

- slow heartbeat
- low blood pressure
- heartbeat problems
- fainting
- tiredness, slowness
- depression (sadness that doesn't go away), anxiety
- decreased interest in sex; impotence
- worsening of congestive heart failure
- worsening of asthma or emphysema

Tell your doctor if you have side effects that do not go away over time, are bothersome, or stop you from taking your medication as directed.

Do other medications interact with topical beta-blockers?

- Beta-blockers may decrease the effectiveness of medications for asthma/emphysema, and chronic obstructive pulmonary disease (COPD).

- If your doctor prescribes a beta-blocker that is available in tablet form and is taken by mouth, use caution due to the possibility for additive effects.

What else should I know about topical beta-blockers?

- Always remember to gently shake the *Betoptic S®* (betaxolol suspension) before every use.

- Use the eye gel preparations the same way as eye ointments.

 ## Warning

- If you have a history of congestive heart failure, asthma, emphysema, diabetes, or depression, discuss the use of these medications with your doctor.

- Be aware of any worsening of symptoms and inform your doctor.

Carbonic Anhydrase Inhibitors

Carbonic anhydrase inhibitors are mild diuretics (water pills) that are sometimes used to treat glaucoma that doesn't respond to other types of medications. They work by decreasing the production of eye fluid. They are effective but have many side effects. They are also available as eye drops.

Oral:

Brand Name	Generic
Daranide®	dichlorphenamide
Diamox®	acetazolamide
Neptazane®	methazolamide

Ophthalmic:

Brand Name	Generic
Trusopt®	dorzolamide

How do I use carbonic anhydrase inhibitors?

The tablets or capsules are taken by mouth one to four times a day, depending on the specific preparation. Take with food to reduce the chance of stomach upset. The eye drops are generally used three times a day. See page 108 for directions on how to use eye drops.

If you miss a dose of this medication, take it as soon as possible. However, if it is almost time for your next dose, skip the missed dose and go back to the dosing schedule. Do not double your dose. It is very important to take your medication exactly as directed by your doctor. NEVER stop taking your prescription medications without talking with your doctor.

What side effects are possible from the use of carbonic anhydrase inhibitors?

Oral:

More Common

- tiredness, slowness, weakness
- loss of appetite and weight loss
- decreased interest in sex; impotence
- depression (sadness that doesn't go away)
- reduced vision
- upset stomach
- vomiting
- diarrhea
- increased uric acid (worsening of gout)

Less Common

- kidney stones
- rash
- blood cell changes

Ophthalmic:

More Common

- bitter taste
- burning, stinging
- sensitivity of eyes to light

Less Common

- dryness of eyes
- headache
- nausea
- unusual tiredness or weakness

Tell your doctor if you have side effects that do not go away over time, are bothersome, or stop you from taking your medication as directed.

Do other medications interact with carbonic anhydrase inhibitors?

- Carbonic anhydrase inhibitors that are taken by mouth may change how other medications work. You should be cautious when using salicylates (anti-inflammatory medications), which may increase the carbonic anhydrase inhibitor levels along with other toxic effects.

- *Dolobid*® (diflunisal) may significantly lower pressure in the eye when given with oral carbonic anhydrase inhibitors.

 # Warning

- If you are allergic to sulfa medications, use caution when taking carbonic anhydrase inhibitors.

- Patients with severe kidney, liver, or lung disease should talk with their doctors before taking any of these agents.

Prostaglandin Analog

Xalatan® (latanoprost) is a new eye drop used to treat glaucoma. This agent will reduce pressure in the eye by helping fluid to drain. This agent is usually used when other agents have not worked.

Brand Name	Generic
Xalatan®	latanoprost

How do I use a prostaglandin analog?

Xalatan® is an eye drop taken one time a day, usually in the evening. See page 108 for directions on how to use eye drops.

If you miss a dose of this medication, take it as soon as possible. However, if it is almost time for your next dose, skip the missed dose and go back to the dosing schedule. Do not double your dose. It is very important to take your medication exactly as directed by your doctor. NEVER stop taking your prescription medications without talking with your doctor.

What side effects are possible from the use of prostaglandin analog?

More Common

- blurred vision
- burning and stinging
- itching
- headache
- sensitivity to light may change the color of the eye to a more brown color

Less Common

- dry eye
- eyelid swelling
- tearing

Tell your doctor if you have side effects that do not go away over time, are bothersome, or stop you from taking your medication as directed.

Do other medications interact with prostaglandin analog?

- *Xalatan*® (latanoprost) will form solid particles with thimerosal (a preservative in many ophthalmic products). Ask your doctor or pharmacist if any of your other eye drops contain thimerosal.

- Use *Xalatan*® 5 to 10 minutes apart from other eye agents that use thimerosal as a preservative.

 ## Warning

You should remove your contact lenses before using the drops. The contact lenses can be put back in your eyes 15 minutes after using *Xalatan*®.

How do I use eye drops?

1. Wash your hands.

2. Tilt your head back or lie down. With one hand, gently pull the lower lid down.

3. If the dropper is separate, squeeze the rubber bulb once while in the bottle to bring liquid into the dropper.

4. Then, holding the dropper or tip of the bottle (if there is no dropper) above the eye, drop the medication inside the lower lid while looking up. Be careful not to touch the dropper or tip of the bottle to the eye or to the fingers.

5. Gently close the eye and look down. Immediately press your forefinger against the inside corner of your eye to prevent the medication from entering the tear duct. Hold your finger there for three to five minutes. This will help to keep the medication in contact with the eye and to decrease absorption into the bloodstream.

6. Replace the dropper or cap tightly, and keep the medication in a dry place. Wash your hands to remove any medication from them, and wash off any medication that may have spilled on your face.

Additional tips:

- If the dropper is separate, always hold it with the tip down.

- Never touch the dropper or tip of the bottle to any surface.

- Never rinse the dropper.

- Never use eye drops that have changed color.

- If you are using more than one kind of drop at the same time, wait 5 to 10 minutes between the different kinds of drops.

How do I use eye ointments and gels?

1. Wash your hands.

2. Remove the cap from the tube.

3. Tilt your head back or lie down. With one hand, gently pull the lower lid down.

4. While looking up, squeeze a small amount of ointment (about 1/4 to 1/2 inch) in a sweeping motion inside the lower lid. Be careful not to touch the tip of the tube to the eye or to your fingers.

5. Close your eye gently and, keeping it closed, roll your eyeball in all directions. Temporary blurring may occur.

6. Replace the cap on the tube. Store the tube in a dry place. Wash your hands to remove any medication from them, and wash off any medication that may have spilled on your face.

Additional tips:

- When opening the tube for the first time, squeeze out the first 1/4 inch and discard, since it may be too dry.

- Never touch the tip of the tube to any surface.

- If you are using more than one kind of ointment at the same time, wait 5 to 10 minutes between different kinds of ointments. Also, if you are using eye drops at the same time as ointments, use the drops first and then the ointment.

- Hold the ointment tube in your hand for a few minutes to warm the ointment and facilitate flow.

Notes

_____

_____

_____

_____

_____

_____

_____

_____

_____

_____

_____

_____

_____

_____

_____

_____

_____

_____

_____

_____

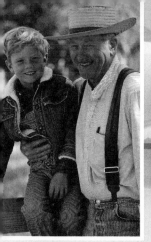

Heartburn, Indigestion and Ulcers

What are heartburn (acid reflux disease), indigestion (dyspepsia), and ulcers (peptic ulcer disease)?

Some of the more common digestive problems are heartburn, indigestion, and ulcers (also known as peptic ulcer disease or PUD).

<u>Indigestion</u> is pain, discomfort, fullness, or bloating associated with eating.

<u>Heartburn</u> sometimes happens when acid from the stomach causes burning and soreness in the lining of the stomach and/or the esophagus (the tube that carries food to the stomach). Symptoms of heartburn are usually a burning feeling in the middle of the chest behind the breastbone after eating. Heartburn may be caused by eating certain foods such as chocolate, fried foods, or foods with tomato. Smoking cigarettes, drinking alcohol, or lying down after eating may also cause heartburn.

<u>Ulcers</u> are sores in the lining of the stomach or small intestine. Ulcers occur when the lining of the stomach or small intestine breaks down due to damage caused by the acid produced by the stomach to digest foods. Most ulcers are caused by an infection called *Helicobacter pylori*. Some ulcers are caused by pain medications, such as aspirin, ibuprofen, or other NSAIDS (see Arthritis and Pain section). Common symptoms are gnawing pain, burning, soreness or an empty feeling in the stomach.

To treat digestive problems, you may need to make changes in your diet and lifestyle and/or take medication. There are five types of medications for indigestion, heartburn, and PUD:

1) medications that decrease acid production, such as *Tagamet*® (cimetidine) and *Prilosec*® (omeprazole)

2) medications that protect the lining of the stomach from acid, such as *Carafate*® (sucralfate)

3) medications that weaken acid, such as antacids

4) antibiotics to treat *H. pylori* infection

5) medications that increase movement of food through the stomach and intestines, such as *Propulsid*® (cisapride) and *Reglan*® (metoclopramide).

Medications that decrease acid production

H2 Antagonists (H2 Blockers)

Special cells in the lining of the stomach make acid to help you digest foods. People with infrequent heartburn or indigestion are best treated with antacids or histamine 2 blockers (H2 blockers) only when they have symptoms. H2 blockers should be used for six to eight weeks to treat an ulcer or for symptoms of frequent heartburn. A small percentage of people with ulcers need to take a smaller dose for up to one year to prevent the symptoms from returning.

Brand Name	Generic
Axid®	nizatidine
Pepcid®	famotidine
Tagamet®	cimetidine
Zantac®	ranitidine

How do I use H2 antagonists (H2 blockers)?

For ulcers, these medications are usually taken once a day at bedtime for 6-8 weeks. Some older people should take smaller doses of these medications than younger people because they can build up if the kidneys have slowed down because of aging. The lower doses are usually *Zantac®* (ranitidine) or *Axid®* (nizatidine) 150 mg; *Tagamet®* (cimetidine) 800 mg; and *Pepcid®* (famotidine) 10 mg to 20 mg. The H2 blockers are best taken before meals, one hour apart from antacids and most other medications.

If you miss a dose of this medication, take it as soon as possible. However, if it is almost time for your next dose, skip the missed dose and go back to the dosing schedule. Do not double your dose. It is very important to take your medication exactly as directed by your doctor. NEVER stop taking your prescription medications without talking with your doctor.

What side effects are possible from the use of H2 antagonists?

Side effects are more common in older adults than in younger adults.

More Common

- confusion
- diarrhea
- dizziness
- muscle aches and pains
- rash

Less Common

- increase in the size of the breast in men (cimetidine)
- decreased interest in sex in men (cimetidine)

Rare

- abnormal blood cells and weakening of the body's defense against disease

Tell your doctor if you have side effects that do not go away over time, are bothersome, or stop you from taking your medication as directed.

Do other medications interact with H2 antagonists?

Tagamet® interacts with many medications, possibly leading to harmful effects. This can usually be prevented by reducing the doses of the following medications.

Tagamet® <u>increases</u> the effects of :

- *Coumadin*® (warfarin)

- *Dilantin*® (phenytoin)

- *Inderal*® (propranolol)

- *Neoral*® and *Sandimmune*® (both brand names of cyclosporine)

- *Procardia*® (nifedipine)

- *Procan*® (procainamide)

- *Quinaglute*® (quinidine)

- *Tegretol*® (carbamazepine)

- *Theo-Dur*® (theophylline)

- *Valium*® (diazepam)

Tagamet® may <u>decrease</u> the absorption of *Nizoral*® (ketoconazole) and *Sporanox*® (itraconazole).

Zantac®, *Axid*®, and *Pepcid*® may also interact with the above-mentioned medications, though to a lesser extent than *Tagamet*®. Check with your doctor or pharmacist for a more complete explanation. Always let your doctor know all of the medications you are taking.

What else should I know about H2 antagonists (H2 blockers)?

- Tell your doctor about any illness that continues for a long time, such as a fever, a cold, or a sore throat.

- Always remember to check with your doctor before taking other medications in combination with H2 blockers. *Never take over-the-counter H2 blockers while you are taking prescription H2 blockers.*

 ## Warning

Talk to your doctor or pharmacist before taking any over-the-counter medications. Some of the over-the-counter medications may contain an H2 blocker which may increase the chance of side effects. Others may contain aspirin or nonsteroidal anti-inflammatory drugs (NSAIDs) that can worsen your stomach problem.

Proton Pump Inhibitors

These medications work by preventing the release of acid in the stomach. These agents are generally used for gastroesophageal reflux disease (GERD) and peptic ulcer disease (PUD).

Brand Name	Generic
Prevacid®	lansoprazole
Prilosec®	omeprazole

How do I use proton pump inhibitors?

Prilosec® (omeprazole) and *Prevacid*® (lansoprazole) are taken once (or twice) daily. Take them in the morning before you eat and before you take other medications (they should be taken on an empty stomach). Swallow the capsules whole; do not crush, open, or chew the capsules.

If you miss a dose of this medication, take it as soon as possible. However, if it is almost time for your next dose, skip the missed dose and go back to the dosing schedule. Do not double your dose. It is very important to take your medication exactly as directed by your doctor. NEVER stop taking your prescription medications without talking with your doctor.

What side effects are possible from the use of proton pump inhibitors?

Rare

- headache
- nausea
- diarrhea
- vomiting
- constipation
- dizziness
- stomach pain
- rash

Tell your doctor if you have side effects that do not go away over time, are bothersome, or stop you from taking your medication as directed.

Do other medications interact with proton pump inhibitors?

Prilosec® increases the effects of:

- *Valium® (diazepam)*
- *Dilantin® (phenytoin)*
- *Coumadin® (warfarin)*
- *Lanoxin® (digoxin)*

Always let your doctor know all of the medications you are taking.

Cytoprotective Agents

Carafate® (sucralfate) and Cytotec® (misoprostol) are agents used to protect the lining of the stomach. Carafate® is especially useful for older people since it causes few side effects, although it can affect the absorption of other medicines. Only Cytotec® prevents ulcers caused by NSAIDs, but diarrhea and stomach pain are common with this medication.

Brand Name	Generic
Carafate®	sucralfate
Cytotec®	misoprostol

How do I use cytoprotective agents?

Carafate® may interfere with the absorption of many medications and should be taken at least two hours apart from other medications (especially antacids). It is usually taken four times a day (one hour before meals and at bedtime) for the treatment of peptic ulcer disease (PUD). You may take Carafate® two times a day if you are on a prevention schedule for PUD. Cytotec® should be taken two to four times a day with meals and at bedtime.

If you miss a dose of this medication, take it as soon as possible. However, if it is almost time for your next dose, skip the missed dose and go back to the dosing schedule. Do not double your dose. It is very important to take your medication exactly as directed by your doctor. NEVER stop taking your prescription medications without talking with your doctor.

What side effects are possible from the use of cytoprotective agents?

Carafate®: constipation.

Cytotec®: diarrhea, stomach pain, or nausea. Taking *Cytotec*® with food may help to ease the side effects.

Tell your doctor if you have side effects that do not go away over time, are bothersome, or stop you from taking your medication as directed.

Do other medications interact with cytoprotective agents?

• *Carafate*® may <u>decrease</u> the absorption of some medications, including *Lanoxin*® and *Lanoxicaps*® (both are brand names of digoxin), *Dilantin*® (phenytoin), *Theo-Dur*® (theophylline), *Cipro*® (ciprofloxacin), and *Sporanox*® (itraconazole).

• Antacids, H2 blockers, and proton pump inhibitors should not be used with *Carafate*®.

• All of these agents should be given at least two hours apart from *Carafate*®.

Acid Neutralizers (Antacids)

Antacids are medications that neutralize (change and weaken) stomach acid. They usually contain combinations of aluminum, calcium, or magnesium. Antacids may be as effective as H2 blockers in the treatment of ulcers, and they have fewer side effects (magnesium–diarrhea; aluminum–constipation). However, antacids need to be taken more frequently than H2 blockers. Simethicone may be added to some combinations to ease flatulence (gas).

Brand Name	Generic
AlternaGEL®, Amphojel®, Basaljel®	aluminum hydroxide
Alka-Mints®, Alkets®, Amitone®, Chooz®, Dicarbosil®, Equilet®, Mallamint® (sugar-free), *Titralac®, Tums®*	calcium carbonate
Phillips' Milk of Magnesia®	magnesium salts
Alka-Seltzer® (effervescent tablet), *Bell/ans®, Bromo-Seltzer®, Citrocarbonate®*	sodium bicarbonate
Losopan®, Riopan®	magaldrate (aluminum hydroxide, magnesium hydroxide sulfate)
Alamag®, Gaviscon® (with alginic acid), *Maalox®* (suspension), *Magnalox®*	aluminum hydroxide, magnesium salts
Marblen®, Mylanta® (chewable tablet and gelcap), *Rolaids®*	calcium carbonate, magnesium salts
Di-Gel® (liquid), *Gelusil®, Kudrox®, Maalox®* Anti-gas/Antacid (chewable tablet), *Mylanta®* (liquid), *Simaal®*	aluminum hydroxide, magnesium salts & simethicone
Titralac® Plus Antacid, *Tums®* Anti-gas/Antacid	calcium carbonate & simethicone
Losopan Plus®, Riopan Plus®	magaldrate & simethicone
Tempo Drops®	calcium carbonate, aluminum hydroxide, magnesium salts & simethicone
Di-Gel® (chewable tablet)	calcium carbonate, magnesium salts & simethicone

How do I use antacids?

For heartburn that happens only once in a while, take antacids as needed. To treat active peptic ulcers, antacids should be taken one and three hours after meals and at bedtime.

Antacids interfere with the absorption of many other medications. Take other medications an hour before or two hours after taking antacids.

If you miss a dose, don't be concerned. Take your next scheduled dose as needed. Do not double your dose.

What side effects are possible from the use of antacids?

- diarrhea (magnesium)
- stomach cramps
- constipation (aluminum or calcium)
- hard feces stuck in the colon (lower part of intestine)
- high magnesium levels (magnesium)

You may take a combination form of aluminum hydroxide and magnesium hydroxide (*Maalox*®, *Mylanta*®, etc.) to reduce the side effects of each type of antacid. Alternating types of antacids can prevent these side effects. For example, giving magnesium hydroxide for one dose, then aluminum hydroxide for the second dose, and so on.

Tell your doctor if you have side effects that do not go away over time, are bothersome, or stop you from taking your medication as directed.

Do other medications interact with antacids?

Antacids interfere with the absorption of many medications, especially antibiotics such as *Achromycin*® (tetracycline), *Lanoxin*® (digoxin), and H2 blockers. Antacids may reduce the effect of *Carafate*® (sucralfate).

What else should I know about antacids?

- Take antacids one hour before or two hours after other medications.

- Liquid antacid preparations are more effective than tablets, but may be less pleasant to take and are less convenient than tablets.

 # Warning

- High doses of antacids taken over a period of weeks or months may cause or worsen high blood pressure, kidney stones, kidney disease, or heart failure.

- Sodium bicarbonate, or baking soda (in *Alka-Seltzer*® and other antacids that bubble and fizz in water), and aspirin should generally not be used, since they are very high in sodium.

- Be sure to tell your doctor if you have any other medical problems.

Antibiotics (Used in Various Combinations)

Recently, doctors have learned that bacteria called *H. pylori* cause peptic ulcer disease in most people. Antibiotics (medicines that fight germs like bacteria) combined with other types of ulcer treatments can kill the bacteria and prevent the ulcer from coming back.

Brand Name	Generic
Achromycin®	tetracycline
Amoxil®	amoxicillin
Biaxin®	clarithromycin
Flagyl®	metronidazole
Pepto-Bismol® (anti-diarrhea medication that is sometimes given with an antibiotic)	bismuth subsalicylate
Polymox®	amoxicillin
Trimox®	amoxicillin

How do I use antibiotics?

Be sure to follow your doctor's directions carefully. It may be necessary to take the medications at different times to avoid drug interactions. Be sure to complete the course of treatment even if you feel better before all the pills are taken. Antibiotics are usually taken with H2 blockers or proton pump inhibitors to treat the ulcer.

If you miss a dose of this medication, take it as soon as possible. However, if it is almost time for your next dose, skip the missed dose and go back to the dosing schedule. Do not double your dose. It is very important to take your medication exactly as directed by your doctor. NEVER stop taking your prescription medications without talking with your doctor.

What side effects are possible from the use of antibiotics?

The side effects that can occur depend on which antibiotic is given and how long the medication is taken. You should know that many patients do not have problem side effects when taking these medications, but there is a possibility for serious side effects in some people. The following is a list of some of the more common side effects of each of the medications. It is not a complete list and you should always tell your doctor if you feel any uncomfortable effects during treatment.

Amoxil®, Polymox®, Trimox® (amoxicillin)

- stomach problems including nausea, vomiting, diarrhea, and skin rashes
- rash
- vaginitis (yeast infection of the vagina)

Let your doctor know if you have had any allergic or bad reactions to amoxicillin, penicillin, or any of the cephalosporin antibiotics in the past.

Report any cases of severe or lasting diarrhea to your doctor because this may be a sign of a serious problem with the intestines.

Pepto-Bismol® (bismuth subsalicylate)

More Common

- harmless darkening of the tongue and stools

Less Common

- hearing problems, including loss of hearing or ringing in the ears
- confusion
- dizziness
- vision problems
- rapid breathing
- headache
- thirstiness
- constipation

Tell your doctor if you have side effects that do not go away over time, are bothersome, or stop you from taking your medication as directed.

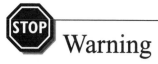

Warning

You should not take *Pepto-Bismol®* if you are allergic to aspirin.

Biaxin® (clarithromycin)

More Common

- headache
- diarrhea
- nausea and stomach pain
- changes in the sense of taste

Rare

- heartbeat problems
- decreased white blood cells
- changes in liver and kidney blood tests

Tell your doctor if you have side effects that do not go away over time, are bothersome, or stop you from taking your medication as directed.

Warning

Report any cases of severe or lasting diarrhea to your doctor because this may be a sign of a serious problem with the intestines.

Flagyl® (metronidazole)

More Common

- dizziness
- nausea
- vomiting
- diarrhea
- loss of appetite
- headache

Less Common

- urine may be discolored to a dark or reddish-brown
- low numbers of certain blood cells
- a taste of metal in the mouth
- sleep problems
- yeast infection (candida) in the vagina
- hives, rash
- fever
- bad response (stomach problems, flushing, headache) after drinking alcohol (beer, wine, whiskey, etc.)
- a furry and/or irritated tongue

Tell your doctor if you have side effects that do not go away over time, are bothersome, or stop you from taking your medication as directed.

 Warning

Avoid all alcoholic beverages (wine, beer, whiskey, etc.) while taking *Flagyl®*.

Achromycin® (tetracycline)

More Common

- diarrhea (mild)
- sensitivity to sunlight with increased risk for sunburn
- nausea

Less Common

- kidney failure
- liver problems
- peeling of the skin and severe skin rash
- soreness and irritation of the throat, pain or difficulty swallowing
- diarrhea (severe)
- vomiting
- vaginitis (yeast infection of the vagina)

Tell your doctor if you have side effects that do not go away over time, are bothersome, or stop you from taking your medication as directed.

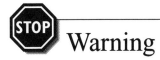 # Warning

If you have kidney disease, be sure that your doctor knows before you take *Achromycin®*, because the dose of medication may need to be reduced.

Do other medications interact with antibiotics?

Amoxil®, Polymox®, Trimox® (amoxicillin)

- *Benemid®* and *Probalan®* (probenecid) may <u>increase</u> the effects of amoxicillin.

- *Zyloprim®* (allopurinol) with amoxicillin may <u>increase</u> the chance of a rash.

Pepto-Bismol® (bismuth subsalicylate)

Pepto-Bismol® <u>increases</u> the effects of:

- *Coumadin®* (warfarin)

- insulin or oral medications for diabetes

- aspirin or aspirin-like medications

Pepto-Bismol® <u>decreases</u> the effects of:

- *Benemid®* and *Probalan®* (probenecid)

- tetracycline (an antibiotic)

Biaxin® (clarithromycin)

Biaxin® increases the effects of:

- *Hismanal®* (astemizole)

- *Coumadin®* (warfarin) and other "blood thinners"

- *Tegretol®* (carbamazepine)

- *Propulsid®* (cisapride)

- *Neoral®* and *Sandimmune®* (cyclosporine)

- *Lanoxin®* (digoxin)

- *Cafergot®*, *Ergomar®*, and *Wigraine®* (ergotamine)

- *Seldane®* (terfenadine)

- *Theo-Dur®*, *Slo-bid®* and *Theolair®* (theophylline)

- *Halcion®* (triazolam)

- *AZT* or *Retrovir®* (zidovudine)

- *Prilosec®* (omeprazole)

The following *increase* the effects of Biaxin®:

- *Orap®* (pimozide)

- *Diflucan®* (fluconazole)

- *Prilosec®* (omeprazole)

 Warning

Many of the drug interactions with *Biaxin®* can cause fatal heartbeat problems. Talk to your doctor before taking any of these medications.

Flagyl® (metronidazole)

Flagyl® may <u>increase</u> *the effects of:*

- alcohol (beer, wine, whiskey, etc.)

- *Antabuse®* (disulfiram)

- *Eskalith®, Lithobid®* and *Lithotabs®* (lithium)

- *Dilantin®* (phenytoin)

- *Coumadin®* (warfarin) and other "blood thinners"

The following may <u>decrease</u> the effects of *Flagyl®*:

- *Luminal®* (phenobarbital)

 # Warning

Do not drink alcohol (beer, wine, whiskey, etc.) during treatment with *Flagyl®*, or for three days after stopping *Flagyl®*, because it can cause stomach pain, nausea, vomiting, headaches, and flushing.

Serious mental effects can occur if *Flagyl®* is taken at the same time as disulfiram. Do not take *Flagyl®* if you have taken disulfiram within two weeks.

Achromycin® (tetracycline)

The following may <u>decrease</u> the effects of *Achromycin®*:

- *Penvee®* K

- *Veetids®*

- *Betapen®-VK* (penicillin)

Achromycin® can <u>increase</u> the effects of:

• *Coumadin®* (warfarin) and other "blood thinners"

The following can <u>decrease</u> the absorption and effects of *Achromycin®*:

• Iron (various over-the-counter)

• *Tagamet®* (cimetidine)

• *Mylanta®*, *Maalox®*, and other products that contain aluminum, calcium, or magnesium (antacids)

 # Warning

Be sure to discard any unused *Achromycin®* (tetracycline). Expired medications can cause severe kidney problems.

Drugs that Increase Movement of Food Through the Digestive System

Propulsid® (cisapride) and *Reglan®* (metoclopramide) are two medications used for the treatment of gastroesophageal reflux disease (GERD). This is a condition in which food and acid from the stomach flow back into the esophagus (the tube that leads to the stomach), causing heartburn and indigestion. By pushing the food along, as well as tightening the ring that separates the stomach from the esophagus, these medications help stop the backflow of food and acid and prevent the uncomfortable symptoms.

Brand Name	Generic
Propulsid®	cisapride
Reglan®	metoclopramide

How do I use Propulsid® and Reglan®?

Propulsid® is available as tablets or in liquid form. It is usually taken four times a day, 15 minutes before each meal, and at bedtime.

Reglan® is available in tablet and syrup forms. It is usually taken four times a day, 30 minutes before each meal, and at bedtime.

What side effects are possible from the use of Propulsid®?

More Common

- headache
- diarrhea
- stomach pain
- nausea
- constipation
- gas
- runny nose
- upper respiratory and viral infection
- pain

Less Common

- indigestion
- urinary tract infection
- fever
- insomnia (trouble sleeping)
- rash
- coughing
- anxiety/nervousness
- joint pain
- vision problems
- itching
- vaginal irritation/soreness

Tell your doctor if you have side effects that do not go away over time, are bothersome, or stop you from taking your medication as directed.

What are the side effects of Reglan®?

More Common

- restlessness
- drowsiness
- tiredness
- weakness
- nausea
- diarrhea

Less Common or Rare

- anxiety and "hyper" feeling
- changes in heartbeat
- confusion
- continuous flow of milk from breasts
- depression (sad feelings that don't go away)
- dizziness
- headache
- increased size of male breasts
- insomnia (trouble sleeping)
- low or high blood pressure
- need to urinate often/leaking urine
- serious allergic reactions (rash, tongue and face swelling, e.g., asthma-like symptoms)
- slow, uncontrolled movement
- stiff muscles
- vision problems

Tell your doctor if you have side effects that do not go away over time, are bothersome, or stop you from taking your medication as directed.

Do other medications interact with Propulsid® and Reglan®?

The following _decrease_ the effects of _Propulsid®_ and _Reglan®_:

- _Atropine®_ (anticholinergic medication)
- _Diflucan®_ (fluconazole)
- _Bellafoline®_ (anticholinergic medication)
- _Pro-Banthine®_ (anticholinergic medication)
- _Quarzan®_
- _Sinemet®_ (levodopa)
- narcotics

Reglan® _decreases_ the effects of:

- _Lanoxin®_ (digoxin)
- _Tagamet®_ (cimetidine)

Reglan® _increases_ the effects of:

- alcohol (beer, wine, whiskey, etc.)
- _Sandimmune®, Neoral®_ (cyclosporine)
- _Sinemet®_ (levodopa)
- _Nardil®, Parnate®_ (MAO inhibitors)

Propulsid® _increases_ the effects of:

- _Zantac®_ (ranitidine)
- _Tagamet®_ (cimetidine)
- _Coumadin®_ (warfarin)

The following _increase_ the effects of _Propulsid®_:

- _Biaxin®_ (clarithromycin)
- _Diflucan®_ (fluconazole)
- _E-Mycin®, Eryc®_ (erythromycin)

- *Nizoral*® (ketoconazole)

- *Sporanox*® (itraconazole)

- *TAO*® (troleandomycin)

 ## Warning

Some drug interactions with *Propulsid*® may cause fatal heartbeat problems. Talk to your doctor before taking any new medication.

Notes

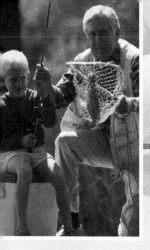

Heart Disease and Chest Pain

What are heart disease (coronary artery disease) and chest pain (angina)?

Heart disease

When a person has coronary artery disease, the vessels that supply blood to the heart are narrowed, limiting the amount of blood and oxygen that reach the heart. The usual cause is a buildup of fatty deposits (also called plaques) on the walls of the arteries. Spasm (sudden closing) of the arteries may also block the vessels.

For the heart to beat and pump blood normally, the heart muscle needs a non-stop supply of oxygen from the blood. If coronary artery disease is not treated, not enough blood can reach the heart. This causes heart damage.

Angina (chest pain)

Angina is chest pain due to coronary artery disease. When the arteries are narrowed or blocked for any reason and the blood flow to the heart cannot increase to meet the need for more oxygen, chest pain may occur.

Not everyone with poor blood supply to the heart has symptoms. Most commonly, a person feels chest pain under the breastbone. Pain may also occur in the left shoulder or down the inside of the left arm, or in the jaw or teeth.

Chest pain is often started by physical activity that lasts no more than a few minutes, and lessens with rest. Some people know how much physical activity will cause episodes of chest pain. Chest pain may start in some people when they exercise right after a meal, walk into the wind, or move from a warm room into cold air.

Treatment for these conditions may include medications, surgery, and changes in lifestyle including losing weight, eating low-fat and low-cholesterol diets, and getting regular exercise. Chest pain may be a sign of worsening heart disease. If untreated, it may lead to a heart attack or death.

Medications used to treat coronary artery disease and chest pain

Nitrates

Nitrates are one of the oldest and most common types of medications used to relieve chest pain. They dilate (open up) the blood vessels in the body, which decreases the amount of work that the heart has to do to pump more blood. Nitrates also dilate the coronary arteries, allowing more blood to flow to the heart. Nitrates also relieve coronary artery spasm.

Brand Name	Generic
Aerosol	
Nitrogard®	nitroglycerin
Nitrolingual®	
Chewable	
Sorbitrate®	isosorbide dinitrate
Ointments	
Nitro-Bid®, Nitrol®	nitroglycerin 2%
Nitrostat®	
Oral	
Dilatrate-SR®, Isonate®	isosorbide dinitrate
Isorbide®, Isordil®	
Nitro-Bid®, Nitrocap T.D.®	nitroglycerin
Nitroglyn®, Nitrolin®	
Nitrong®, Nitrospan®, Nitrostat®	
Sorbitrate®	isosorbide dinitrate
Sublingual	
Isordil®	isosorbide dinitrate
Nitrostat®	nitroglycerin
Sorbitrate®	isosorbide dinitrate
Transdermal	
Deponit®, Nitrodisc®	nitroglycerin
Nitro-Dur®	
Transderm-Nitro®	

How do I use nitrates?

There are many different forms of nitrates, and all have two basic effects: reducing chest pain or preventing heart attack. You should sit or lie down when taking forms of nitrate under the tongue, in a spray, held in the cheek, or chewed to minimize the sudden drop in blood pressure that can occur right after taking the drug.

Some nitrates are taken daily to prevent chest pain and some nitrates may be taken either when chest pain begins or right before it is likely to occur.

If you miss a dose of this medication, take it as soon as possible. However, if it is almost time for your next dose, skip the missed dose and go back to the dosing schedule. Do not double your dose. It is very important to take your medication exactly as directed by your doctor. NEVER stop taking your prescription medications without talking with your doctor.

Nitrate tablets taken under the tongue

These tablets are usually the first choice to relieve symptoms of common angina. They work rapidly, providing relief within minutes, and are simple to use. They can also be taken before exercise or hard physical activity to prevent angina or to relieve it after it occurs.

These tablets spoil over time and become unusable. They should be kept in their original containers with tightly fitting caps. Keep them out of sunlight. **Throw away any tablets more than six months old.**

All of these forms are kept in the mouth until dissolved and not swallowed so that they enter into the bloodstream quickly.

These tablets come in many different strengths. A dose may be repeated about every five minutes until there is relief, but no more than three tablets should be taken in a 15-minute period. If this dose fails to control symptoms, contact your doctor immediately or go to the nearest hospital or emergency room.

Aerosols

Aerosols are sprayed onto or under the tongue. They must never be inhaled. These work as well as the under-the-tongue tablets and can be taken for the same reasons. Aerosols are simple to use and are most used by people who have difficulty dissolving the under-the-tongue form of the drug.

Chewable and oral tablets

Chewable nitroglycerin provides rapid relief. The long-acting oral forms are chewed and swallowed and released slowly from the stomach. Chewable nitroglycerin tablets are used to prevent angina. Isosorbide dinitrate and nitroglycerin are both effective, although their dosages are different.

Ointments

Nitroglycerin ointments are longer acting than the under-the-tongue or aerosol forms, but ointments can be messy, and some people find them difficult to apply. The dose is usually measured in inches of ointment from a tube every four to six hours and applied to the skin almost anywhere on the trunk or upper arms. These ointments are used to prevent angina.

Transdermal patches

Transdermal patches are easy to apply and are used daily to prevent angina. They are self-sticking and are placed on the skin, almost anywhere on the trunk or upper arms. Changing where you place the patch each time will help to prevent skin irritation. Like ointments, they are absorbed through the skin. These patches are usually left on for 12 to 14 hours, then removed. They are used to prevent angina.

What side effects are possible from the use of nitrates?

- increased heartbeat
- headaches – may occur at first (these can be severe but usually go away after a few days or weeks). In the meantime, aspirin or acetaminophen can provide relief.
- flushing
- light-headedness upon standing – may lead to fainting
- rash – may occur with ointments or patches

- dizziness
- swelling

Tell your doctor if you have side effects that do not go away over time, are bothersome, or stop you from taking your medication as directed.

Do other medications interact with nitrates?

Nitrates may intensify the blood pressure-lowering effects of antihypertensives and other antianginal medications. Nitrates may also cause low blood pressure when combined with *Viagra*® (sildenafil).

Calcium Channel Blockers

These agents are used widely and are effective among older people for the treatment of hypertension (high blood pressure). They relax blood vessels, increasing the supply of blood and oxygen to the heart while reducing the work load of the heart.

Calcium channel blockers dilate (expand) large blood vessels and decrease blood pressure. They allow more blood to reach the heart and reduce the work load of the heart.

Some calcium channel blockers are excellent medications for angina and generally cause few problems in older people. Some are used when there is a need to treat both high blood pressure and angina. In this way, one medication may be enough for two problems.

Brand Name	Generic
Adalat® CC	nifedipine
Calan® SR	verapamil
Cardene®	nicardipine
Cardene® SR	nicardipine
Cardizem® CD	diltiazem
Dilacor® XR	diltiazem
DynaCirc®	isradipine
Isoptin® SR	verapamil
Norvasc®	amlodipine
Plendil®	felodipine
Procardia® XL	nifedipine
Sular®	nisoldipine
Verelan®	verapamil

How do I use calcium channel blockers?

Calcium channel blockers are taken every day, either once a day or up to three times a day. Do not crush or chew pills before swallowing.

If you miss a dose of this medication, take it as soon as possible. However, if it is almost time for your next dose, skip the missed dose and go back to the dosing schedule. Do not double your dose. It is very important to take your medication exactly as directed by your doctor. NEVER stop taking your prescription medications without talking with your doctor.

What side effects are possible from the use of calcium channel blockers?

More Common

- leg swelling, especially with *Adalat®*, *Procardia®* (both brand names of nifedipine)
- constipation
- low blood pressure
- slow heartbeat with *Cardizem®* (diltiazem) and *Calan®* (verapamil)

Less Common

- nausea, diarrhea
- rash
- abnormal heartbeat
- dizziness
- headache

Tell your doctor if you have side effects that do not go away over time, are bothersome, or stop you from taking your medication as directed.

Do other medications interact with calcium channel blockers?

The calcium channel blockers may *increase* the blood pressure-lowering effects of other high blood pressure medications (antihypertensives) or medications for angina/shortness of breath (antianginal).

They may also *increase* the effects of *Theo-Dur®* (theophylline), *Tegretol®* (carbamazepine), *Sandimmune®* and *Neoral®* (cyclosporine), and *Lanoxin®* (digoxin).

Cardizem® (diltiazem) and *Calan®* (verapamil) slow the heart rate and may *increase* the effects of *Lanoxin®* (digoxin) and beta-blockers.

Tagamet® (cimetidine) may *increase* the effects of calcium channel blockers.

What else can calcium channel blockers be used for?

Calcium channel blockers can also be used for high blood pressure or to reduce the number of migraine headaches.

What else should I know about calcium channel blockers?

- Take your medication every day as directed by your doctor even if you feel well.

- These medications need to be taken daily to prevent angina symptoms and to prevent a heart attack.

- If you are taking a sustained-release tablet or capsule, be certain not to crush or chew the medication.

Beta-Blockers

Beta-blockers slow the heart rate and decrease blood pressure. They work by blocking the system in our body that responds to stress or danger by quickly elevating blood pressure. The beta-blockers are useful in patients who have fast heart rates, chest pain, and migraine headaches, as well as for those who have had a heart attack.

Beta-blockers such as *Lopressor®* and *Toprol-XL®* (metoprolol), *Tenormin®* (atenolol), and *Sectral®* (acebutolol) affect specific areas in the heart; they may be better for people with long-term lung disease or poor circulation. Beta-blockers such as *Visken®* (pindolol), *Trasicor®* (oxprenolol), and *Sectral®* (acebutolol) cause less slowing of the heart and may be better for people with a slow heartbeat.

Beta-blockers, such as *Inderal®* (propranolol) and *Lopressor®* and *Toprol-XL®* (metoprolol), tend to produce more side effects – such as colorful dreams, hallucinations (unreal visions), nightmares, depression (sadness that doesn't go away), drowsiness, and confusion – than most other commonly used antihypertensive medications.

Some beta-blockers are very effective in controlling angina. Studies have shown that patients treated with beta-blockers following a heart attack can live longer. Beta-blockers are well tolerated by most patients, although they may cause more problems for older people.

Like the calcium channel blockers, beta-blockers decrease the heart's need for oxygen, slow the heart rate, and lower blood pressure. By doing so, they reduce the heart's work load and chest pain.

Brand Name	Generic
Betaloc®	metoprolol
Betapace®	sotalol
Blocadren®	timolol
Cartrol®	carteolol
Corgard®	nadolol
Inderal®	propranolol
Kerlone®	betaxolol
Levatol®	penbutolol
Lopressor®	metoprolol
Normodyne®	labetalol
Sectral®	acebutolol
Sotacor®	sotalol
Tenormin®	atenolol
Trandate®	labetalol
Trasicor®	oxprenolol
Visken®	pindolol
Zebeta®	bisoprolol

How do I use beta-blockers?

Some long-acting beta-blockers are taken only once a day, while others need to be taken more frequently. They come in tablet or capsule form.

If you miss a dose of this medication, take it as soon as possible. However, if it is almost time for your next dose, skip the missed dose and go back to the dosing schedule. Do not double your dose. It is very important to take your medication exactly as directed by your doctor. NEVER stop taking your prescription medications without talking with your doctor.

What side effects are possible from the use of beta-blockers?

More Common

- heart failure
- low blood pressure
- slow heartbeat
- dizziness
- weakness
- tiredness
- loss of interest in sex; impotence

Less Common

- colorful dreams
- depression (sadness that doesn't go away)
- stomach upset
- rashes
- leg pain when walking
- shortness of breath

Tell your doctor if you have side effects that do not go away over time, are bothersome, or stop you from taking your medication as directed.

Do other medications interact with beta-blockers?

- other high blood pressure medications

- *Tagamet*® (cimetidine)

- *Quinora*® (quinidine) may *increase* the effects of beta-blockers.

- *Rifadin*® (rifampin), *Solfoton*® (phenobarbital), nonsteroidal anti-inflammatory medications (NSAIDs), and thyroid hormones may *decrease* the effects of beta-blockers.

What else can beta-blockers be used for?

Helping to prevent heart attacks, correcting irregular heartbeats, preventing migraine headaches, and treating tremors (shakiness).

What else should I know about beta-blockers?

Older people with any of the following conditions should consult their doctors to be sure they can take beta-blockers safely:

- depression (sadness that doesn't go away)

- heart failure

- asthma

- emphysema

- bronchitis

- diabetes

- coronary obstructive pulmonary disease (COPD)

- poor circulation

Warning

- Beta-blockers may worsen the symptoms of asthma, emphysema, bronchitis, or chronic obstructive pulmonary disease (COPD).

- Beta-blockers may hide the symptoms of low blood sugar (hypoglycemia) and may cause problems for people with diabetes.

- Beta-blockers may worsen the symptoms of poor circulation (peripheral vascular disease).

- Beta-blockers may cause or worsen depression (sadness that doesn't go away) and cause tiredness.

Never stop taking beta-blockers suddenly, except on the advice of a doctor; doing so may worsen or uncover symptoms of coronary artery disease or cause high blood pressure.

Notes

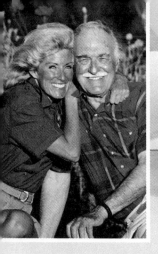

Heart Failure

What is congestive heart failure?

Heart failure (also known as congestive heart failure) occurs when the heart cannot pump enough blood to meet the body's needs. Heart failure can result from coronary artery disease (narrowing of the blood vessels called arteries that supply blood to the heart), a past heart attack, high blood pressure, heart valve disease, and infection of the heart or heart valves. In people with heart failure, the heart keeps working but not as well as it should. When you have heart failure, blood backs up in the veins, fluid fills the lungs, and swelling of the legs and ankles occurs. Patients may be weak, have problems breathing, develop swollen legs or ankles, and gain weight. Treatment of heart failure includes rest, proper diet, and medication.

Medications used to treat heart failure

Lanoxicaps®/Lanoxin® (digoxin)

Lanoxicaps® and Lanoxin® have been used for many years to treat heart failure, as well as abnormal heart rhythm, known as atrial fibrillation. Lanoxicaps® and Lanoxin® increase the power of each heartbeat and slow a heartbeat that is too fast.

Brand Name	Generic
Lanoxicaps®	digoxin
Lanoxin®	digoxin

How do I use Lanoxicaps®/Lanoxin®?

Lanoxicaps® and *Lanoxin®* are generally taken once each day or once every other day. When used to treat heart failure, doses can generally be kept low, and little adjustment is needed.

Varying amounts of digoxin may need to be taken on different days to get the right blood level.

If you miss a dose of this medication, take it as soon as possible. However, if it is almost time for your next dose, skip the missed dose and go back to the dosing schedule. Do not double your dose. It is very important to take your medication exactly as directed by your doctor. NEVER stop taking your prescription medications without talking with your doctor.

What side effects are possible from the use of Lanoxicaps®/Lanoxin®?

- loss of appetite
- nausea
- vomiting
- diarrhea
- stomach pain
- dizziness
- slow heartbeat
- tiredness
- weakness
- confusion
- problems with vision
- fainting
- high blood sugar
- gout

Tell your doctor if you have side effects that do not go away over time, are bothersome, or stop you from taking your medication as directed.

Do other medications interact with Lanoxicaps®/Lanoxin®?

The following drugs may _increase_ the effects of digoxin levels in the blood:

- *Achromycin®* (tetracycline)
- *Adalat®* (nifedipine)
- *Calan®* (verapamil)
- *Cordarone®* (amiodarone)
- diuretics (water pills)
- *Ery-Tab®* (erythromycin)
- *Isoptin®* (verapamil)
- *Midamor®* (amiloride)
- *PCE®* (erythromycin)
- *Plaquenil®* (hydroxychloroquine)
- *Procardia®* (nifedipine)
- *Quinidex®* (quinidine)
- *Quinora®* (quinidine)
- (reserpine)
- *Rythmol®* (propafenone)
- *Sandimmune®* (cyclosporine)
- *Sporanox®* (itraconazole)
- *Vascor®* (bepridil)
- *Xanax®* (alprazolam)

The following medications may _decrease_ the effects of digoxin:

- *Azulfidine®* (sulfasalazine)
- *Carafate®* (sucralfate)
- *Colestid®* (colestipol)
- *Dilantin®* (phenytoin)
- *Gaviscon®* (antacid)
- *Imodium®* (antidiarrheal preparation)

- *Kaopectate® (kaolin and pectin)*
- *Maalox®* (antacid)
- *Metamucil® (psyllium)*
- *Mylanta®* (antacid)
- *Neo-Tabs®* (neomycin)
- *Pepto-Bismol®* (antidiarrheal preparations)
- *Questran®* (cholestyramine)
- *Rifadin®* (rifampin)
- *Solfoton®* (phenobarbital)

What else should I know about Lanocaps®/Lanoxin®?

- Be sure to remind your doctor that you are taking digoxin when any new medications are prescribed. Ask your pharmacist about any possible interactions when you buy over-the-counter (non-prescription) medications.

- Hypokalemia (low levels of the mineral potassium in the blood) can lead to digoxin toxicity and the development of abnormal heart rhythms. If you are taking diuretics (water pills), which lower potassium levels, be sure to follow your doctor's instructions about diet and the use of potassium supplements (potassium in a tablet or powder form).

Loop Diuretics (water pills)

Loop diuretics are often used to treat heart failure. They work by getting rid of salt and water from the body through urine. Lowering the amount of fluid in your body reduces the amount of work the heart has to do. Loop diuretics are effective, easy to take, and they have few side effects. Their doses may need to be changed with changes in weather, diet, and the function of the heart.

Brand Name	Generic
Bumex®	bumetanide
Demadex®	torsemide
Edecrin®	ethacrynic acid
Lasix®	furosemide

How do I use loop diuretics?

These medications are taken once a day, usually in the morning (to avoid nighttime trips to the bathroom). If your physician prescribes a loop diuretic twice a day, it is recommended that one dose be taken early in the morning and the second dose be taken early in the afternoon (again, to avoid waking up during the night to go to the bathroom). Loop diuretics may sometimes be used on alternate days or even just three days per week. If you have to urinate frequently, you may want to take your medication after returning home from activities outside the house.

If you miss a dose of this medication, take it as soon as possible. However, if it is almost time for your next dose, skip the missed dose and go back to the dosing schedule. Do not double your dose. It is very important to take your medication exactly as directed by your doctor. NEVER stop taking your prescription medications without talking with your doctor.

What side effects are possible from the use of loop diuretics?

- hypokalemia (low potassium)
- changes in levels of sodium, chloride, bicarbonate, and other important minerals called electrolytes
- dehydration (loss of too much water from the body)
- low blood pressure
- muscle cramps
- rash
- weakness, tiredness

Tell your doctor if you have side effects that do not go away over time, are bothersome, or stop you from taking your medication as directed.

Do other medications interact with loop diuretics?

- Loop diuretics may lead to a low potassium level when they are taken with corticosteroids.

- Loop diuretics taken with lithium may increase the levels of lithium.

- Caution should be taken when loop diuretics are combined with digoxin. Digoxin toxicity occurs most commonly in the presence of low potassium levels.

What else can loop diuretics be used for?

Loop diuretics are also used to reduce leg swelling, high blood pressure, and decrease fluid that builds up with kidney failure.

What else should I know about loop diuretics?

The level of electrolytes (minerals in the blood), especially that of potassium, should be checked occasionally by a blood test.

 # Warning

- Electrolyte changes may cause muscle cramps, weakness, confusion, irritability, nausea, vomiting, or abnormal heart rhythms. Report any of these conditions to your doctor.

- Some people taking loop diuretics also need potassium supplements; eating potassium-rich foods such as citrus fruits, tomatoes, bananas, watermelon, and potatoes can also help. Most people who take both

ACE (angiotensin converting enzyme) inhibitors and diuretics do not take potassium supplements.

- Older people often become dehydrated. That may result in low blood pressure, especially upon standing. Low blood pressure can cause light-headedness, falling, or even fainting.

- Talk to your doctor before using salt substitutes. Salt substitutes may contain potassium which can cause problems with some medications.

Angiotensin Converting Enzyme (ACE) Inhibitors

ACE inhibitors relax blood vessels and open up the arteries, veins, or both. They reduce the work required by the heart and help to lower blood pressure. These medications have been shown to help patients with heart failure live longer.

ACE inhibitors are also made in combination with various diuretics. For most older people, it is better to take the medications separately so that you receive the best dose of each medication.

Brand Name	Generic
Accupril®	quinapril
Altace®	ramipril
Capoten®	captopril
Lotensin®	benazepril
Monopril®	fosinopril
Prinivil®	lisinopril
Univasc®	moexipril
Vasotec®	enalapril
Zestril®	lisinopril

How do I use angiotensin converting enzyme (ACE) inhibitors?

Capoten® (captopril) is generally taken from two to three times a day. All others are taken once or twice daily at higher doses. The absorption of *Capoten®* is affected by food, so it should be taken one hour before or two hours after meals. This is not a concern with the other ACE inhibitors.

If you miss a dose of this medication, take it as soon as possible. However, if it is almost time for your next dose, skip the missed dose and go back to the dosing schedule. Do not double your dose. It is very important to take your medication exactly as directed by your doctor. NEVER stop taking your prescription medications without talking with your doctor.

What side effects are possible from the use of ACE inhibitors?

The first dose of an ACE inhibitor can lower your blood pressure greatly, while your body is getting used to the drug. Side effects may include:

More Common

- change in the sense of taste
- a lasting dry cough
- headache
- dizziness
- increased potassium levels
- rash, itchy skin
- low blood pressure (hypotension) with the first dose taken
- tiredness

Less Common

- flushing and swelling of face, lips, tongue, arms, and legs
- changes in how well the kidneys work
- blood disorders/anemias (low number of blood cells)

Tell your doctor if you have side effects that do not go away over time, are bothersome, or stop you from taking your medication as directed.

Do other medications interact with ACE inhibitors?

• Allopurinol may increase the chance of unwanted side effects.

• Diuretics may increase the action of ACE inhibitors.

• Any other medication for high blood pressure (antihypertensive medication) may cause low blood pressure when taken with an ACE inhibitor.

• Potassium-sparing diuretics and potassium supplements may cause increased potassium levels that can be dangerous.

What else should I know about angiotensin converting enzyme (ACE) inhibitors?

• Report any sore throat, fever, sores, cough, or swelling to your doctor immediately.

• Do not use salt substitutes without checking with your doctor because some may contain potassium.

Warning

- Never take potassium-sparing diuretics or potassium supplements when on ACE inhibitors without first checking with your doctor.

- Since dizziness, light-headedness, or fainting may occur with the first dose, a friend or family member should watch you when you take your first dose, and you should avoid any strenuous activity for several hours afterward. You should see your doctor often and have your blood pressure checked several times during the first few weeks of therapy.

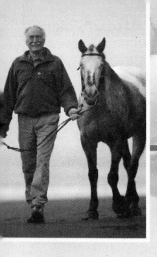

High Blood Pressure

What is high blood pressure (hypertension)?

The heart pumps blood through blood vessels to bring oxygen and nutrients to the body. As blood flows through the vessels, it puts pressure on the walls of the blood vessels. Blood pressure is the measurement of this pressure against the walls. The higher the pressure, the harder the heart has to work.

When your blood pressure is checked, two numbers are given. The top number (systolic pressure) is measured when the heart beats and the bottom number (diastolic pressure) is measured when the heart is at rest. For example, 120/80 mm Hg is an average blood pressure reading.

If you have high blood pressure (hypertension), this means that your pressure is higher than what is normal. For older adults, high blood pressure is defined as having a top number (systolic pressure) greater than 140 mm Hg and/or a bottom number (diastolic pressure) greater than 90 mm Hg on at least two measurements.

High blood pressure is not a normal condition of getting older.

The following may increase your blood pressure:

• obesity

• large amounts of salt in food

• stress

• tension

• nervousness

High blood pressure is known as the "silent killer" because the patient does not experience any obvious symptoms. If high blood pressure is left untreated, it may lead to other complications such as a heart attack, stroke, or kidney disease.

It is important to get your blood pressure checked regularly. If you are diagnosed with high blood pressure, there are many ways you can be treated. Treatment of high blood pressure may include changes in diet (such as eating less salt), losing weight, getting regular exercise, quitting smoking, and taking medication.

Medications used to treat high blood pressure

Many different medications are used to treat high blood pressure. Many doctors begin therapy with a water pill (diuretic). If the patient's blood pressure remains high or if there are other problems, such as chest pain or heart failure, another medication may be substituted for or added to the diuretic. Your doctor will work with you to find the medication that works best for you.

Diuretics (Water Pills)

Diuretics help the kidneys get rid of salt and water through urine. This lowers the amount of fluid in the blood and widens the blood vessels, which lowers blood pressure.

Diuretics are commonly used to treat high blood pressure. There are two main types of diuretics. Some of these water pills cause potassium (one of the important minerals in the blood known as electrolytes) to be removed from the body through the urine. These are called potassium-depleting diuretics. Other diuretics cause the kidneys to keep potassium. They are called potassium-sparing diuretics. Some water pills combine both potassium-depleting and potassium-sparing diuretics. Sometimes they are combined with other types of antihypertensive (high blood pressure) medications to make them easier to take, although such combinations are usually not the best choice for older people.

A diuretic is often the drug of first choice for the control of simple high blood pressure in older people. Diuretics are effective and easy to take, and they have few side effects.

Potassium-depleting diuretics (causes potassium loss)

HydroDIURIL® (hydrochlorothiazide) is the most frequently prescribed diuretic for treating high blood pressure in older people. It works well, even at low doses, and many older people will not need to take extra potassium when using it. *HydroDIURIL®* may be used in heart failure patients but is more likely used in the treatment of high blood pressure.

Brand Name	Generic
Anhydron®	cyclothiazide
Bumex®	bumetanide
Demadex®	torsemide
Diucardin®	hydroflumethiazide
Diurese®	trichlormethiazide
Diuril®	chlorothiazide
Edecrin®	ethacrynic acid
Enduron®	methyclothiazide
Exna®	benzthiazide
HydroDIURIL®	hydrochlorothiazide

Chart continues on following page

Brand Name	Generic
Hydromox®	quinethazone
Hygroton®	chlorthalidone
Lasix®	furosemide
Lozol®	indapamide
Naturetin®	bendroflumethiazide
Renese®	polythiazide
Zaroxolyn®	metolazone

How do I use potassium-depleting diuretics?

These medications are usually taken only once a day, usually in the morning (to avoid nighttime trips to the bathroom). People who have to urinate a lot may want to take them after returning home from activities outside the house.

If you miss a dose of this medication, take it as soon as possible. However, if it is almost time for your next dose, skip the missed dose and go back to the dosing schedule. Do not double your dose. It is very important to take your medication exactly as directed by your doctor. NEVER stop taking your prescription medications without talking with your doctor.

What side effects are possible from the use of potassium-depleting diuretics?

- low levels of potassium in the blood
- gout (a type of arthritis)
- changes in levels of sodium, chloride, bicarbonate, and other important minerals
- increased blood sugar
- dehydration (loss of too much water from the body)

- rash
- low blood pressure
- weakness, tiredness
- muscle cramps

Tell your doctor if you have side effects that do not go away over time, are bothersome, or stop you from taking your medication as directed.

Do other medications interact with potassium-depleting diuretics?

- If taken with potassium-depleting diuretics, corticosteroids may lower potassium levels.

- Low potassium from diuretics may cause *Lanoxin*® (digoxin) toxicity.

- Diuretics may also <u>increase</u> the level of lithium in the blood.

What else can potassium-depleting diuretics be used for?

Potassium-depleting diuretics are also used for reducing leg swelling, kidney failure, heart failure, kidney stones, and liver disease.

What else should I know about potassium-depleting diuretics?

You will need to take your medication daily to control your blood pressure to prevent heart attacks, strokes, or kidney failure.

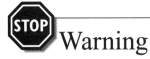

Warning

- The level of electrolytes (minerals in the blood), especially that of potassium, should be checked occasionally by a blood test. Electrolyte changes may cause muscle cramps or weakness, confusion, irritability, nausea, vomiting, or abnormal heartbeat. Report any of these conditions to your doctor.

- Older people easily become dehydrated (lose too much water) from these medications. This may result in low blood pressure or light-headedness upon standing. Low blood pressure can cause light-headedness, falling, or fainting.

- Some people taking loop diuretics also need potassium supplements; eating potassium-rich foods such as citrus fruits, tomatoes, bananas, watermelon, and potatoes can also help. Most people who take both ACE (angiotensin converting enzyme) inhibitors and diuretics do not take potassium supplements.

- Talk to your doctor before using salt substitutes. Salt substitutes may contain potassium which can cause problems with some medications.

Potassium-Sparing Diuretics (no potassium loss)

These diuretics are rarely used alone. They are often used in combination to prevent low potassium levels.

Brand Name	Generic
Aldactone®	spironolactone
Dyrenium®	triamterene
Midamor®	amiloride

How do I use potassium-sparing diuretics ?

The potassium-sparing diuretics are generally taken one to four times a day.

If you miss a dose of this medication, take it as soon as possible. However, if it is almost time for your next dose, skip the missed dose and go back to the dosing schedule. Do not double your dose. It is very important to take your medication exactly as directed by your doctor. NEVER stop taking your prescription medications without talking with your doctor.

What are some possible side effects from the use of potassium-sparing diuretics?

- high potassium levels
- decreased interest in sex
- leg swelling
- dizziness
- low blood pressure

Tell your doctor if you have side effects that do not go away over time, are bothersome, or stop you from taking your medication as directed.

Do other medications interact with potassium-sparing diuretics?

- If taken with potassium-sparing diuretics, nonsteroidal anti-inflammatory medications (NSAIDs) may *increase* potassium levels or worsen kidney problems.

- Potassium supplements may be life-threatening due to *increased* potassium levels.

- ACE inhibitors may cause high potassium levels.

What else should I know about potassium-sparing diuretics?

- Increased potassium levels may also be seen in older patients who have kidney disease or who have diabetes.

- Blood potassium levels should be monitored periodically.

- You will need to take your medication daily to control your blood pressure to prevent heart attacks, strokes, or kidney failure.

 # Warning

- Individuals taking these medications should avoid salt substitutes and large amounts of foods high in potassium such as citrus fruits, bananas, watermelon, and potatoes unless directed by your doctor.

- Consult with your doctor before taking any potassium supplements or any other medication, such as an ACE inhibitor.

Mixed Diuretics

A mixed diuretic is a combination of a potassium-sparing and a potassium-depleting diuretic (a water pill). Such medications can be used to treat heart failure, but they are more likely to be used in the treatment of high blood pressure.

Combinations of potassium-depleting and potassium-sparing medications:

Brand Name	Generic
Aldactazide®	spironolactone & hydrochlorothiazide
Dyazide®, *Maxzide*®	triamterene & hydrochlorothiazide
Moduretic®	amiloride & hydrochlorothiazide

How do I use mixed diuretics?

Take once or twice a day as directed by your physician.

If you miss a dose of this medication, take it as soon as possible. However, if it is almost time for your next dose, skip the missed dose and go back to the dosing schedule. Do not double your dose. It is very important to take your medication exactly as directed by your doctor. NEVER stop taking your prescription medications without talking with your doctor.

What side effects are possible from the use of mixed diuretics?

- dryness of mouth
- increased thirst
- muscle cramps or pain
- loss of appetite
- dizziness
- low blood pressure
- high or low potassium levels
- gout (a form of arthritis)

- increased blood sugar
- dehydration (loss of too much water)

Tell your doctor if you have side effects that do not go away over time, are bothersome, or stop you from taking your medication as directed.

What else should I know about mixed diuretics?

- These are combination medications and therefore have all the interactions and special warnings for both types of diuretics.

- You will need to take your medication daily to control your blood pressure to prevent heart attacks, strokes, or kidney failure.

Diuretics Combined with Other Agents

These medications are a combination of a potassium-depleting diuretic and another drug. See the sections on diuretics and the other medications separately for more information.

Some other antihypertensive medications lower blood pressure by relaxing the blood vessels, and the potassium-depleting diuretic helps to lower blood pressure by reducing the amount of water in the body. This combination medication may be prescribed so that you will have fewer pills to take each day.

Diuretics combined with other antihypertensives*:

Brand Name	Generic
Capozide®	hydrochlorothiazide & captopril
Inderide®	hydrochlorothiazide & propranolol
Minizide®	hydrochlorothiazide & prazosin
Vaseretic®	hydrochlorothiazide & enalapril

*There are many such combination products; a complete listing is beyond the scope of this book. Four of the more commonly prescribed products are listed.

Beta-Blockers

Beta-blockers slow the heart rate and decrease blood pressure by blocking the system in our bodies that raises blood pressure quickly in times of stress. These are useful in patients who have fast heartbeats, chest pain, migraine headaches, or those who have had a heart attack.

Beta-blockers such as Lopressor® and Toprol-XL® (both brand names of metoprolol), Tenormin® (atenolol), and Sectral® (acebutolol) affect specific areas in the heart; they may be preferred for people with lung disease or poor circulation. Other beta-blockers, such as Visken® (pindolol), Trasicor® (oxprenolol), and Sectral® cause less slowing of the heart and may be better for people with a slow heartbeat.

Beta-blockers such as *Inderal*® (propranolol) and *Lopressor*® and *Toprol-XL*®, are more likely to cause side effects, such as colorful dreams, hallucinations (seeing strange, unreal visions), nightmares, depression (sadness that doesn't go away), drowsiness, and confusion, than most other commonly used beta-blockers.

Some beta-blockers are very effective in controlling angina (chest pain). Studies have shown that treating patients with beta-blockers after a heart attack can help them to live longer. Beta-blockers do not cause problem side effects in most patients, although beta-blockers may cause more problems for older people.

Beta-blockers decrease the heart's need for oxygen, slow the heart pulse, and lower blood pressure. By doing so, they reduce the heart's workload and thus, chest pain (angina).

Brand Name	Generic
Betaloc®	metoprolol
Betapace®	sotalol
Blocadren®	timolol
Cartrol®	carteolol
Corgard®	nadolol
Inderal®	propranolol
Kerlone®	betaxolol
Levatol®	penbutolol
Lopressor®	metoprolol
Normodyne®	labetalol
Sectral®	acebutolol
Tenormin®	atenolol

Table continues on following page

Brand Name	Generic
Toprol-XL®	metaprolol
Trandate®	labetalol
Trasicor®	oxprenolol
Visken®	pindolol
Zebeta®	bisoprolol

How do I use beta-blockers?

Some long-acting beta-blockers are taken only once a day; others need to be taken more often. They come in tablet or capsule form. In general, they may be taken with most other medications.

If you miss a dose of this medication, take it as soon as possible. However, if it is almost time for your next dose, skip the missed dose and go back to the dosing schedule. Do not double your dose. It is very important to take your medication exactly as directed by your doctor. NEVER stop taking your prescription medications without talking with your doctor.

What side effects are possible from the use of beta-blockers?

More Common

- heart failure
- low blood pressure
- slow heartbeat
- dizziness
- weakness
- tiredness
- loss of interest in sex; impotence

Less Common

- colorful dreams
- depression (sadness that doesn't go away)
- stomach upset
- rashes
- leg pain when walking
- shortness of breath

Tell your doctor if you have side effects that do not go away over time, are bothersome, or stop you from taking your medication as directed.

Do other medications interact with beta-blockers?

The following may *increase* the effects of beta-blockers:

- other high blood pressure medications
- *Tagamet*® (cimetidine)
- *Quinora*® (quinidine)

The following may *decrease* the effects of beta-blockers:

- *Rifadin*® (rifampin)
- nonsteroidal anti-inflammatory drugs (NSAIDs)
- *Solfoton*® (phenobarbital)
- thyroid hormones

What else can beta-blockers be used for?

Beta-blockers are also used for relieving chest pain (angina), helping to prevent additional heart attacks in heart attack patients, correcting an irregular heartbeat, preventing the number of migraine headaches, and treating tremors.

What else should I know about beta-blockers?

Older people with any of the following conditions should consult their doctor to be sure they can take beta-blockers safely:

- depression (sadness that doesn't go away)

- heart failure

- asthma

- emphysema

- chronic bronchitis

- diabetes

- chronic obstructive pulmonary disease (COPD)

- poor circulation

 Warning

- You will need to take your medication daily to control your blood pressure to prevent heart attacks, strokes, or kidney failure.

- Beta-blockers may worsen symptoms of asthma, emphysema, bronchitis, or chronic obstructive pulmonary disease (COPD).

- Beta-blockers may hide the symptoms of low blood sugar (hypoglycemia), which may cause problems for people with diabetes.

- Beta-blockers may worsen the symptoms of poor circulation (peripheral vascular disease).

- Beta-blockers may cause or worsen depression (sadness that doesn't go away) and cause tiredness.

- Never stop taking beta-blockers suddenly, except on the advice of a doctor; doing so may worsen or lead to symptoms of coronary artery disease.

ACE Inhibitors

ACE (angiotensin converting enzyme) inhibitors relax and open the blood vessels, which lowers blood pressure and increases the supply of blood and oxygen to the heart.

ACE inhibitors are often combined with various water pills (diuretics). Your doctor may prescribe these medications separately, so that the dose of each medication can be adjusted for each person.

Brand Name	Generic
Accupril®	quinapril
Altace®	ramipril
Capoten®	captopril
Lotensin®	benazepril
Monopril®	fosinopril
Prinivil®	lisinopril
Univasc®	moexipril
Vasotec®	enalapril
Zestril®	lisinopril

How do I use ACE inhibitors?

ACE inhibitors come in tablet or capsule form. *Capoten*® (captopril) is generally taken from two to three times a day. All others are taken once or twice daily at higher doses. The absorption of *Capoten*® is affected by food so it should be taken one hour before or two hours after meals. This is not a concern with other ACE inhibitors.

If you miss a dose of this medication, take it as soon as possible. However, if it is almost time for your next dose, skip the missed dose and go back to the dosing schedule. Do not double your dose. It is very important to take your medication exactly as directed by your doctor. NEVER stop taking your prescription medications without talking with your doctor.

What side effects are possible from the use of ACE inhibitors?

More Common

- changes in the taste of food
- headache
- rash, itchy skin
- dizziness
- lasting dry cough
- tiredness
- increased potassium levels
- low blood pressure (hypotension) when the first dose is taken

Less Common

- blood disorders/anemia (low number of red blood cells)
- flushing and swelling of face, lips, tongue, arms, and legs
- changes in how well the kidneys work

Do other medications interact with ACE inhibitors?

- When taken with ACE inhibitors, *Zyloprim*® (allopurinol) may _increase_ chances of a skin reaction.

- Diuretics may _increase_ the actions of ACE inhibitors.

- Potassium-sparing diuretics or potassium supplements may _increase_ potassium levels.

- Any medication for high blood pressure (antihypertensives) may cause low blood pressure when taken with an ACE inhibitor.

What else should I know about ACE inhibitors?

• Report any sore throat, fever, sores, cough, or swelling to your doctor.

• You will need to take your medication daily to control your blood pressure to prevent heart attacks, strokes, or kidney failure.

 # Warning

• Talk to your doctor before using salt substitutes. Salt substitutes may contain potassium which can cause problems with some medications. Older people taking this medication should avoid excess amounts of foods high in potassium such as citrus fruits, bananas, watermelon, and potatoes, unless directed by your doctor.

• Since dizziness, light-headedness, or fainting may occur with the first dose of an ACE inhibitor, you should have a friend or family member supervise you for your first dose, and you should avoid any strenuous activity for several hours afterward. You should see your doctor frequently and have your blood pressure checked several times during the first few weeks of taking this type of medication.

Angiotensin II Inhibitors

These agents block a substance in the body that causes the blood vessels to tighten (constrict) which raises blood pressure. When the substance is blocked, the blood vessels are able to relax, allowing blood and oxygen to pass through them more easily. This helps to lower blood pressure.

Brand Name	Generic
Avapro®	irbesartan
Cozaar®	losartan
Diovan®	valsartan

How do I use angiotensin II inhibitors?

Angiotensin II inhibitors come in tablet or capsule form. *Cozaar*® (losartan) is usually given once or twice daily, with or without food. *Diovan*® (valsartan) and *Avapro*® (irbesartan) are usually given once daily.

Angiotensin II inhibitors are often combined with water pills (diuretics). Your doctor may prescribe these medications separately, so that the dose of each medication can be adjusted for each person.

If you miss a dose of this medication, take it as soon as possible. However, if it is almost time for your next dose, skip the missed dose and go back to the dosing schedule. Do not double your dose. It is very important to take your medication exactly as directed by your doctor. NEVER stop taking your prescription medications without talking with your doctor.

What side effects are possible from the use of angiotensin II inhibitors?

More Common

- headache
- dizziness
- tiredness
- insomnia (trouble sleeping)
- diarrhea
- upset stomach (indigestion, sour stomach)
- high potassium levels
- swelling of legs or feet

Less Common

- cough
- fever
- gout (a type of arthritis)
- back pain
- stuffy nose, sore and swollen sinuses
- unsteadiness upon standing

Tell your doctor if you have side effects that do not go away over time, are bothersome, or stop you from taking your medication as directed.

Do other medications interact with angiotensin II inhibitors?

- Diuretics may *increase* the actions of angiotensin II inhibitors.

- Potassium-sparing diuretics or potassium supplements may *increase* potassium levels.

What else should I know about angiotensin II inhibitors?

- Report any hoarseness, swelling of the face, mouth, or hands, or trouble swallowing to your doctor.

- You will need to take your medication daily to control your blood pressure to prevent heart attacks, strokes, or kidney failure.

 # Warning

- Do not take any potassium-sparing diuretics or potassium supplements without first checking with your doctor.

- Since dizziness or light-headedness may occur with the first dose, have a friend or family member watch you, and avoid any hard physical activity for several hours afterwards.

Calcium Channel Blockers

These agents are used in older patients as treatment for hypertension. They relax blood vessels, increasing the supply of blood and oxygen to the heart while reducing the workload of the heart.

Some medications are used for angina and generally cause few problems in older people. Some are used when there is a need to treat both high blood pressure and angina. In this way, one medication may be enough to treat two problems.

Brand Name	Generic
Adalat® CC	nifedipine
Calan® SR	verapamil
Cardene®	nicardipine
Cardene® SR	nicardipine
Cardizem® CD	diltiazem
Dilacor® XR	diltiazem
DynaCirc®	isradipine
Isoptin® SR	verapamil
Norvasc®	amlodipine
Plendil®	felodipine
Procardia® XL	nifedipine
Sular®	nisoldipine
Verelan®	verapamil

How do I use calcium channel blockers?

Calcium channel blockers are taken every day. Some are taken once a day and others are taken up to three times a day. Do not crush or chew these pills before swallowing.

If you miss a dose of this medication, take it as soon as possible. However, if it is almost time for your next dose, skip the missed dose and go back to the dosing schedule. Do not double your dose. It is very important to take your medication exactly as directed by your doctor. NEVER stop taking your prescription medications without talking with your doctor.

What side effects are possible from the use of calcium channel blockers?

More Common

- leg swelling (especially with *Adalat® CC* and *Procardia® XL*, both brand names of nifedipine)
- constipation (especially with *Calan® SR, Isoptin® SR*, and *Verelan®*, all brand names of verapamil)
- low blood pressure
- slow heartbeat (*Cardizem®, Calan®*)

Less Common

- nausea, diarrhea
- rash
- heartbeat problems
- dizziness
- headache

Tell your doctor if you have side effects that do not go away over time, are bothersome, or stop you from taking your medication as directed.

Do other medications interact with calcium channel blockers?

- Calcium channel blockers may _increase_ the blood pressure-lowering effects of other high blood pressure medications (antihypertensive) or medications for chest pain (antianginal).

- The calcium channel blockers may _increase_ the effects of Theo-Dur® (theophylline), Tegretol® (carbamazepine), Lanoxin® (digoxin), and Sandimmune® and Neoral® (both are brand names of cyclosporine).

- Diltiazem and verapamil in combination with Lanoxin® (digoxin) or beta-blockers may slow the heartbeat.

- Tagamet® (cimetidine) may _increase_ the effects of calcium channel blockers.

What else can calcium channel blockers be used for?

Calcium channel blockers are also used for angina (chest pain), heart beat problems, or to reduce the frequency of migraine headaches.

What else should I know about calcium channel blockers?

- If you are taking a sustained-release tablet or capsule (something named SR, CD, XL, etc.), do not crush or chew the medication.

- Remember that medications for your high blood pressure are not a cure. You will need to take your medication daily to control your blood pressure to prevent heart attacks, strokes, and kidney failure.

Centrally Acting Agents

These medications relax the blood vessels in the body, so that blood passes through them more easily. There are two centrally acting agents that are commonly used: clonidine and methyldopa. Both cause serious side effects in the elderly and are not first choice agents.

"▲" Indicates medications that are generally not recommended for use in older people. Do not stop taking these medications unless directed by your doctor. They may be required under special circumstances. Talk to your doctor to see if this medication is right for you.

Brand Name	Generic
▲ *Aldomet*®	methyldopa
Catapres®	clonidine

How do I use centrally acting agents?

Catapres® (clonidine) is available as a tablet, to be taken from one to three times a day. *Catapres*® is also available in the form of a transdermal (skin) patch that is changed once a week. Applying a patch once per week may be easier for older persons than swallowing the tablet every day.

• The patch should be applied to a clean, dry area of skin on your upper arm or chest, avoiding areas with hair, cuts, or skin irritations.

• The patch should remain in place during showering, bathing, or swimming. If the patch becomes loose, cover it with adhesive tape.

• Apply a new patch if it becomes too loose or falls off.

• Change the patch once a week, applying the new patch to a different site than the previous one to prevent skin irritations.

Aldomet® (methyldopa) is taken once a day at bedtime and then increased to twice daily. It is also available in a liquid form. The centrally acting agents are not affected by food and can be taken with most other medications.

If you miss a dose of this medication, take it as soon as possible. However, if it is almost time for your next dose, skip the missed dose and go back to the dosing schedule. Do not double your dose. It is very important to take your medication exactly as directed by your doctor. NEVER stop taking your prescription medications without talking with your doctor.

What side effects are possible from the use of Catapres®?

More Common

- dry mouth
- constipation
- drowsiness
- headache
- dizziness
- light-headedness upon standing

Less Common

- decreased appetite
- nervousness, agitation, insomnia
- nausea
- heartbeat problems
- weight gain
- rash, hives, skin irritation
- heart failure
- colorful dreams and nightmares
- decreased interest in sex
- impotence

(The transdermal patch causes side effects similar to but less intense than those caused by the tablets.)

What side effects are possible from the use of Aldomet®?

More Common

- drowsiness
- constipation
- headache
- dry mouth
- weakness
- dark urine
- nausea
- light-headedness upon standing

Less Common

- rash
- fever
- heartbeat problems
- decreased interest in sex
- low blood counts

Rare

- anemia
- jaundice (yellowing of skin and the whites of the eye)
- hepatitis (a liver problem)

Tell your doctor if you have side effects that do not go away over time, are bothersome, or stop you from taking your medication as directed.

Do other medications interact with centrally acting agents?

- Antidepressants may reduce the effectiveness of *Catapres*®.

- Withdrawal (rebound) hypertension on stopping *Catapres*® may be worse in people who are also taking beta-blockers.

- *Aldomet*® taken with *Haldol*® (haloperidol) may cause restlessness, changes in your walk pattern, and increase drowsiness.

- Side effects of *Sinemet*® (levodopa) may be increased by *Aldomet*®.

- Blood pressure-lowering effects of *Aldomet*® may also be increased by *Sinemet*®.

- When *Aldomet*® and lithium are taken together, blood levels of lithium may increase.

- When combined with *Orinase*® (tolbutamide), *Aldomet*® may increase the blood sugar-lowering effects of *Orinase*®.

What else can centrally acting agents be used for?

Catapres® is also used to lessen the symptoms that can occur in people trying to quit the use of alcohol (beer, wine, whiskey, etc.), medications, or tobacco. It is also used to treat menopausal hot flashes, Tourette's syndrome, high blood pressure emergencies, and to prevent migraine headaches.

What else should I know about centrally acting agents?

- Never stop *Catapres®* therapy abruptly, except on the advice of a doctor.

- Remember that while using *Aldomet®*, your urine may appear darker. Tell your doctor if you develop lasting flu-like symptoms with tiredness, fever, and joint pain, or if the whites of your eyes become yellowish (jaundice).

You will need to take your medication daily to control your blood pressure to prevent heart attacks, strokes, and kidney failure.

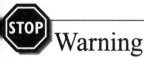 Warning

- *Aldomet®* is not recommended for most older people because it can cause drowsiness, depression, and unsteadiness when standing.

- Since these medications may make you unsteady on your feet, you may be at risk for a fall which can lead to a broken bone. If you have a history of falling, be sure to tell your doctor. Your doctor may be able to change your medication to reduce your risk of falling.

Vasodilators

Vasodilators work by relaxing blood vessels throughout the body so that blood passes through them more easily. This helps to lower blood pressure. Vasodilators are not usually the first choice in older people since they may cause dizziness or light-headedness in persons getting up from a sitting or lying down position. However, your doctor will help decide if a vasodilator is right for you.

Brand Name	Generic
Apresoline®	hydralazine
Cardura®	doxazosin
Hytrin®	terazosin
Rogaine®	minoxidil
Minipress®	prazosin

How do I use vasodilators?

Vasodilators may be taken from one to four times each day. Your doctor will let you know how many times a day to take your medication.

If you miss a dose of this medication, take it as soon as possible. However, if it is almost time for your next dose, skip the missed dose and go back to the dosing schedule. Do not double your dose. It is very important to take your medication exactly as directed by your doctor. NEVER stop taking your prescription medications without talking with your doctor.

What side effects are possible from the use of Minipress®, Cardura®, or Hytrin®?

More Common

- dizziness, light-headedness (especially when getting up from a sitting or lying-down position with the first dose)
- drowsiness
- lack of energy

Less Common

- dry mouth
- nervousness
- loss of bladder control
- increased heartbeat

- leg or feet swelling
- headache

What side effects are possible from the use of Apresoline®?

More Common

- headache
- diarrhea
- loss of appetite
- nausea
- increased heartbeat
- leg or feet swelling

Less Common

- constipation
- dizziness, light-headedness
- flushing of the face
- watering of the eyes
- stuffy nose
- lupus (a reaction that can cause skin rash and damage to the kidneys and other body organs)

What side effects are possible from the use of Rogaine®?

More Common

- increase in hair growth (usually on the face, arms, and back)
- increased heartbeat
- weight gain (more than five pounds)
- bloating
- leg or feet swelling

Less Common

- chest pain
- shortness of breath
- tingling of the hands, feet, or face
- headache

Tell your doctor if you have side effects that do not go away over time, are bothersome, or stop you from taking your medication as directed.

Do other medications interact with vasodilators?

The blood pressure-lowering effect may be increased if minoxidil is taken with a water pill (diuretic) or another high blood pressure medication.

What else can vasodilators be used for?

Cardura® (doxazosin), *Minipress®* (prazosin) and *Hytrin®* (terazosin) are all used for reducing the symptoms of blocked urination, the feeling of having to urinate suddenly, and nighttime urination in men with the prostate problem called benign prostatic hypertrophy (BPH).

A liquid form of *Rogaine®* (minoxidil) is used for stimulating regrowth of hair in patients with male-pattern baldness.

Apresoline® (hydralazine) is also used for treating congestive heart failure.

What else should I know about vasodilators?

- Be careful when taking your first dose. You may have a fainting spell within the first 90 minutes of taking your medication.

- Getting up slowly may lessen any dizziness or light-headedness you might feel after the first dose.

- If you feel dizzy, lie down so that you do not faint.

- To help prevent dizziness, be careful during exercise or hot weather and limit the amount of alcohol (beer, wine, whiskey, etc.) you drink.

- You will need to take your medication daily to control your blood pressure to prevent heart attacks, strokes, and kidney failure.

Since these medications may cause drowsiness, be careful when driving or working with machines.

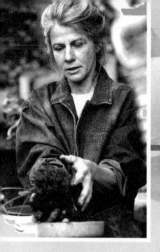

Irregular Heartbeats

What are irregular heartbeats (arrhythmias)?

Arrhythmias are irregular heartbeats. People with arrhythmias have heartbeats that are too slow or too fast. Arrhythmias can cause the heart to work less effectively. There are many kinds of arrhythmias. Some types need treatment, and some do not. If medication is needed, it works best when it is prescribed for the specific type of arrhythmia involved. Some of these medications can also be used for other purposes, such as heart failure or high blood pressure.

Medications used to treat arrhythmias

Lanoxicaps®/Lanoxin® (digoxin)

Lanoxicaps® and *Lanoxin®* are used for abnormal heart rhythms. This is a condition in which the heart does not beat at the right speed, such as the condition called atrial fibrillation (abnormal heart rhythm in the upper part of the heart called the atrium). *Lanoxicaps®* and *Lanoxin®* increase the power of each heartbeat. They also slow a heartbeat that is too fast.

Brand Name	Generic
Lanoxicaps®	digoxin
Lanoxin®	digoxin

How do I use Lanoxicaps®/Lanoxin®?

Lanoxicaps® and *Lanoxin®* are generally taken only once a day. Some older people may be able to take it every other day. Sometimes it is necessary to take different doses on different days to get the right amount of medication in the blood.

If you miss a dose of this medication, take it as soon as possible. However, if it is almost time for your next dose, skip the missed dose and go back to the dosing schedule. Do not double your dose. It is very important to take your medication exactly as directed by your doctor. NEVER stop taking your prescription medications without talking with your doctor.

What side effects are possible from the use of Lanoxicaps®/Lanoxin®?

Tell your physician if you experience any of the following:

- loss of appetite
- tiredness
- nausea
- weakness
- vomiting
- confusion
- diarrhea

- vision problems
- stomach pain
- faintness
- dizziness
- palpitations (irregular heartbeat)
- slow heartbeat

Tell your doctor if you have side effects that do not go away over time, are bothersome, or stop you from taking your medication as directed.

Do other medications interact with Lanoxicaps®/Lanoxin®?

The following medications may *increase* the effects of digoxin levels in the blood:

- *Achromycin*® (tetracycline)
- *Adalat*® (nifedipine)
- *Calan*® (verapamil)
- *Cordarone*® (amiodarone)
- diuretics (water pills)
- *Ery-Tab*® (erythromycin)
- *Isoptin*® (verapamil)
- *Midamor*® (amiloride)
- *PCE*® (erythromycin)
- *Plaquenil*® (hydroxychloroquine)
- *Procardia*® (nifedipine)
- *Quinidex*® (quinidine)
- *Quinora*® (quinidine)
- (reserpine)
- *Rythmol*® (propafenone)
- *Sandimmune*® (cyclosporine)
- *Sporanox*® (itraconazole)
- *Vascor*® (bepridil)
- *Xanax*® (alprazolam)

The following medications may *decrease* the effects of digoxin:

- *Azulfidine*® (sulfasalazine)
- *Carafate*® (sucralfate)
- *Colestid*® (colestipol)
- *Dilantin*® (phenytoin)
- Gaviscon® (antacid)
- *Imodium*® (antidiarrheal preparation)

- *Kaopectate*® (kaolin & pectin)
- *Maalox*® (antacid)
- *Metamucil*® (psyllium)
- *Mylanta*® (antacid)
- *Neo-Tabs*® (neomycin)
- *Pepto-Bismol*®, *Imodium*® (antidiarrheals)
- *Questran*® (cholestyramine)
- *Rifadin*® (rifampin)
- *Solfoton*® (phenobarbital)

What else should I know about Lanoxicaps®/Lanoxin®?

Be sure to remind your doctor that you are taking *Lanoxicaps*® or *Lanoxin*® when any new medications are prescribed. Ask your pharmacist about any possible interactions when buying over-the-counter (non-prescription) medications.

 # Warning

- Hypokalemia (low potassium) can lead to digoxin toxicity and the development of heart rhythm disturbances. If you are taking diuretics (water pills), which lower potassium levels, be sure to follow your doctor's instructions regarding diet and the use of potassium supplements.

- You should have your *Lanoxin*® blood levels checked periodically.

Beta-Blockers

Beta-blockers have many uses. One of their uses is to slow the heartbeat. Beta-blockers also prevent arrhythmias in people who are prone to abnormal heart rhythms, especially after a heart attack. Beta-blockers decrease the heart's need for oxygen, slow the heart rate, and lower blood pressure.

Some beta-blockers are very good at controlling heart-related chest pain. Some studies show that patients treated with beta-blockers following a heart attack may live longer. Beta-blockers are well tolerated by most patients, although they are more problematic for older people.

Different beta-blockers have different effects. For example, some beta-blockers, such as *Lopressor*® (metoprolol), *Toprol-XL*® (metoprolol), *Sectral*® (acebutolol), and *Tenormin*® (atenolol), are more heart selective, mainly affecting the heart rather than other organs. As a result, they may be better for people who also have lung disease or poor circulation. Some beta-blockers, such as *Visken*® (pindolol), *Trasicor*® (oxprenolol), and *Sectral*® (acebutolol), cause less slowing of the heart.

Brand Name	Generic
Betapace®	sotalol
Blocadren®	timolol
Cartrol®	carteolol
Corgard®	nadolol
Inderal®	propranolol
Inderal LA®	propranolol
Kerlone®	betaxolol
Levatol®	penbutolol
Lopressor®	metoprolol
Normodyne®	labetalol
Sectral®	acebutolol
Tenormin®	atenolol
Toprol-XL®	metoprolol
Trandate®	labetalol
Trasicor®	oxprenolol
Visken®	pindolol
Zebeta®	bisoprolol

How do I use beta-blockers?

Some long-acting beta-blockers are taken only once a day. Others need to be taken more frequently. They come in tablet or capsule form.

If you miss a dose of this medication, take it as soon as possible. However, if it is almost time for your next dose, skip the missed dose and go back to the dosing schedule. Do not double your dose. It is very important to take your medication exactly as directed by your doctor. NEVER stop taking your prescription medications without talking with your doctor.

What side effects are possible from the use of beta-blockers?

More Common

- heart failure
- low blood pressure
- slow heartbeat
- dizziness
- weakness
- tiredness
- loss of interest in sex; impotence

Less Common

- colorful dreams
- depression
- stomach upset
- rashes
- leg pain when walking
- shortness of breath

Tell your doctor if you have side effects that do not go away over time, are bothersome, or stop you from taking your medication as directed.

Do other medications interact with beta-blockers?

The following medications may *increase* the effects of beta-blockers:

- high blood pressure medications
- *Quinaglute® Dura-Tabs* (quinidine)
- *Tagamet®* (cimetidine)

The following medications may _decrease_ the effects of beta-blockers:

- nonsteroidal anti-inflammatory medications (NSAIDs)
- _Rifadin_® (rifampin)
- _Solfoton_® (phenobarbital)
- thyroid hormones

What else can beta-blockers be used for?

Beta-blockers are also used to treat high blood pressure, heart attack (myocardial infarction), chest pain (angina), migraine headaches, and mitral valve prolapse syndrome.

What else should I know about beta blockers?

Older people with any of the following conditions should talk with their doctors to be sure they can take beta-blockers safely:

- depression (sadness that doesn't go away)
- heart failure
- asthma
- emphysema
- bronchitis
- diabetes
- chronic obstructive pulmonary disease (COPD)
- poor circulation

Warning

- Beta-blockers may worsen symptoms of lung disease, especially asthma.

- Beta-blockers may also hide the symptoms of low blood sugar (hypoglycemia). Thus, they may cause problems for people with diabetes.

- Beta-blockers may worsen the symptoms of poor circulation (peripheral vascular disease).

- Beta-blockers may also cause or worsen depression and cause tiredness.

- Do not stop taking beta-blockers suddenly, except on the advice of a physician. Doing so may worsen or uncover symptoms of coronary artery disease (angina, chest pain), or cause high blood pressure.

Antiarrhythmics

There are many different types of medications, called "antiarrhythmics" as a group, that are used to prevent or control abnormal heart rhythms. These medications work by changing the electrical conduction through the heart. Doctors must choose the type of medication carefully according to the type of abnormal heart rhythm and the reason why it's happening.

"▲" Indicates medications that are <u>generally not recommended</u> for use in older people. Do not stop taking these medications unless directed by your doctor. They may be required under special circumstances. Talk to your doctor to see if this medication is right for you.

Brand Name	Generic
▲ *Norpace®*	disopyramide
Cardioquin®	quinidine
Cordarone®	amiodarone
Ethmozine®	moricizine
Mexitil®	mexiletine
Procan® SR	procainamide
Pronestyl®	procainamide
Quinaglute® Dura-Tabs	quinidine
Tambocor®	flecainide
Tonocard®	tocainide

Many of these medications cause side effects. It may be necessary for some patients to tolerate some of the side effects because abnormal heart rhythms can be life-threatening and medications must be continued. On the other hand, a switch from one medication to another may reduce the severity of side effects. The doses of these medications are very important and must be matched to each patient's needs.

All of the information about these medications cannot be included in this book. However, there are several important points that you should know.

What else should I know about antiarrhythmics?

- Never stop or change the dose of an antiarrhythmic without first talking with your doctor. If you are about to run out of your medication, contact your pharmacist immediately.

- See your doctor regularly in case the dose of your medication needs to be adjusted.

- If you feel light-headed, develop palpitations (a feeling of rapid or irregular heartbeat), pass out (syncope), or feel like you're about to pass out, contact your doctor immediately.

- Never start or stop any medication without asking your doctor. Other medications may change the amount of the antiarrhythmic in your blood. Always tell your doctor and pharmacist about all the medications you are taking.

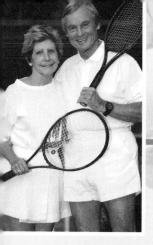

Irritable Bowel Syndrome

What is irritable bowel syndrome?

Irritable bowel syndrome (IBS) affects the stomach and intestines. It is sometimes called "spastic colon" or "colitis" and is common among older people. People with IBS have digestive systems that can be very sensitive to stress, diet, medications, and hormones. IBS symptoms include constipation, diarrhea, or a change back and forth between constipation and diarrhea. Stomach pain, bloating, and cramping may also occur. Treatment for IBS is different for each person. If a type of food can be pinpointed as the cause, it should not be eaten. If stress worsens IBS symptoms, the person should try to reduce stress. If constipation is a problem, regular exercise and eating a diet high in fiber may help. For some people, bulk-forming laxatives may be used as directed by their doctor.

Medications used to treat irritable bowel syndrome

Anticholinergic Antispasmodic Agents

Anticholinergic antispasmodic agents are often prescribed for IBS, but unfortunately, no studies show these medications to be effective. Their action is to slow down the movement of the intestines. These agents may be used for short periods of time but not for long-term treatment of IBS. Their side effects are more common and more harsh in older people, so these medications should rarely, if ever, be used.

"▲" indicates medications that are <u>generally not recommended</u> for use in older people. Do not stop taking these medications unless directed by your doctor. They may be required under special circumstances. Talk to your doctor to see if this medication is right for you.

Brand Name	Generic
▲ Anaspaz®	hyoscyamine
▲ Atropine®	atropine
▲ Bentyl®	dicyclomine
▲ Cantil®	mepenzolate
▲ Cystospaz®	hyoscyamine
▲ Donnatal®	belladonna
▲ Levsin®	hyoscyamine
▲ Pro-Banthine®	propantheline
▲ Quarzan®	clidinium
▲ Robinul®	glycopyrrolate
▲ Transderm Scop®	scopolamine

What side effects are possible from the use of anticholinergic antispasmodic agents?

More Common

• dry mouth

• rapid heartbeat

• widened pupils of the eye

- constipation
- blurred vision
- problems emptying urine from the bladder

Less Common

- flushing
- restlessness, irritability
- fever
- difficulty swallowing
- rash
- seeing strange, unreal visions
- nausea
- light-headedness
- vomiting
- confusion

Tell your doctor if you have side effects that do not go away over time, are bothersome, or stop you from taking your medication as directed.

Do other drugs interact with anticholinergic agents?

Anticholinergics may _decrease_ the effects of:

- *Sinemet®* (levodopa)

Anticholinergics may _increase_ the effects of:

- narcotics
- antipsychotics
- antihistamines
- cyclic antidepressants

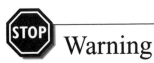 Warning

These agents should be used for short term only. Use carefully if you have any of the following conditions:

- urinary problems or an enlarged prostate
- heart failure
- dementia (Alzheimer's disease)
- glaucoma
- dizziness
- low blood pressure
- severe ulcerative colitis (a serious condition that affects the colon, causing diarrhea that may contain blood)
- liver disease
- kidney disease
- asthma and/or allergies

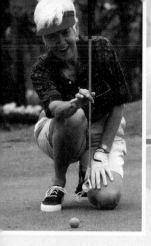

Osteoporosis

What is osteoporosis?

Osteoporosis is a disease that causes bones to become thin, weak, and brittle. It is common among older people and affects one in four women over age 50. It is important to prevent osteoporosis because it is a major cause of fractures in the spine, hip, and wrist. The disease develops over a period of many years, usually silently without causing any pain. Eventually, if it is not treated, the bones thin out and weaken and can break with only a minor injury. One out of every two women over the age of 50 will have an osteoporosis-related fracture in their lifetime.

In younger people new bone is formed to replace old bone. After age 35, more bone is lost than gained. At menopause the bone loss accelerates for three to five years and then continues at a lower rate. The bone loss continues throughout life but doesn't cause problems for women until well after menopause (the time when women stop having their menstrual periods and levels of estrogen, the female sex hormone, fall). Although the reason why osteoporosis develops is not fully understood, most believe it is related to changing hormone levels, hereditary factors, lack of calcium in the diet, and low levels of physical activity.

Women are much more likely to get osteoporosis than men. Women who are fair and have small frames (such as white and Asian women), women who have a family history of osteoporosis, smokers, those who have taken medications such as thyroid, steroids and seizure medications, and women who had early menopause are more likely to get osteoporosis. Treatment often includes changes in diet, regular weight-bearing exercise (like walking), and medication.

Medications used to treat osteoporosis

Estrogen preparations

Estrogen supplements replace the hormone estrogen that is normally made by a woman's body before menopause. Estrogen replacement helps to prevent bone loss. Estrogen reduces the risk of broken bones most effectively when started just after menopause and continued for long periods of time (greater than five years). Benefits appear to be lost a short time after stopping estrogen therapy. However, estrogen treatment for osteoporosis and other conditions, such as protection of the heart and blood vessels, can be of benefit even if started more than 10 years after the start of menopause.

Estrogen should be used in combination with a program of regular weight-bearing exercise, adequate calcium intake, and adequate vitamin D intake.

Brand Name	Generic
Climara® (transdermal patch) Estrace® (tablet, vaginal cream) Estraderm® (transdermal patch) Vivelle® (transdermal patch)	estradiol
Estratab® (tablet) Menest® (tablet)	estrogen, esterified
Ogen® (tablet) Ortho-Est® (tablet)	estropipate
Premarin® (tablet, vaginal cream)	estrogen, conjugated
Premphase® (tablet) Prempro®	conjugated estrogen and medroxyprogesterone

How do I use estrogen preparations?

One of the most commonly used estrogen medications is *Premarin®* (conjugated estrogen). Estrogen is generally taken in pill form, although a transdermal (skin patch) preparation and a vaginal cream are available. Estrogen is usually taken in pill form every day or daily for the first 21 to 25 days of the month. If you still have a uterus, you will need to take a progestin with the estrogen to prevent cancer in the lining of the uterus (endometrial cancer). In women with a uterus, progestins like *Provera®* (medroxyprogesterone acetate) are given daily or for two weeks of every month. If you have had a hysterectomy (removal of the uterus), you will not need to take progestins.

If you miss a dose of this medication, take it as soon as possible. However, if it is almost time for your next dose, skip the missed dose and go back to the dosing schedule. Do not double your dose. It is very important to take your medication exactly as directed by your doctor. NEVER stop taking your prescription medications without talking to your doctor.

What side effects are possible from the use of estrogen?

More Common

- nausea
- fullness and tenderness in the breasts
- swelling caused by salt and water buildup in the body
- menstrual bleeding

Less Common

- increased risk of gallstones
- increased risk of blood clots that could result in deep thrombosis or stroke in some patients
- worsening of migraine headaches
- worsening of endometriosis (a painful overgrowth of the tissue that lines the uterus)
- endometrial cancer
- increased interest in sex
- diarrhea

Uncertain

• increased risk of breast cancer (study results disagree)

Tell your doctor if you have side effects that do not go away over time, are bothersome, or stop you from taking your medication as directed.

What else can estrogen be used for?

Estrogen can also be used for vaginal swelling and soreness with bleeding, itching, or dryness; post-menopausal symptoms in women, such as hot flashes; leaking urine (incontinence) in post-menopausal women; Alzheimer's disease; and prevention of heart and blood vessel disease in post-menopausal women; certain cancers in both men and women.

Do other medications interact with estrogen?

Rifabutin® (rifampin) or *Dilantin*® (phenytoin) <u>decrease</u> the effects of estrogen. Estrogen may <u>increase</u> the effects of corticosteroids. Estrogen may <u>decrease</u> the effect of *Coumadin*® (warfarin).

What else should I know about estrogen?

• The risk of endometrial cancer is increased by the use of estrogen alone in females with an intact uterus (females that have not had a hysterectomy). You should use a progestin like *Provera*® in addition to estrogen to prevent this, if you have not had a hysterectomy.

• Tell your doctor if you have a history of breast cancer, a fibroid uterus, endometriosis, gall bladder disease, or blood clots. Estrogen can make these conditions worse. Your doctor can determine if estrogen is right for you.

• Men and women over 65 years of age should have at least 1500 mg of elemental calcium daily. You can get this from calcium in your diet or from calcium supplements. Talk to your doctor or pharmacist for advice on calcium supplements.

• To absorb calcium you need vitamin D. Some people do not get enough vitamin D from their diet. Talk to your doctor or pharmacist to see if you need to take a vitamin D supplement or a multivitamin.

 ## Warning

Do not use estrogen if you have a history of liver disease, breast cancer, pulmonary embolism (a blood clot in the lungs), vascular thrombosis (blood clot), or unexplained vaginal bleeding.

Evista® (raloxifene)

Evista® (raloxifene) is the first of a new type of estrogen-like medications called selective estrogen receptor modulators (SERMs). The key word in this long, scientific name is *selective*, because this medication affects only some parts of the body that estrogen affects, but not others. For example, *Evista®* affects bone, but does not have the effects of estrogen on the breast or uterus. As a result of these differences, *Evista®* gives women only some of the benefits of estrogen, but also has fewer side effect problems than seen with estrogen.

Evista® is used only to prevent osteoporosis in women after menopause. It does not prevent hot flashes the way that estrogen does. Although *Evista®* helps build bones, it does not work as well as estrogen and it is not yet known if raloxifene can prevent broken bones. *Evista®* may be a good choice for some women because it does not have some of the problem side effects of estrogen. *Evista®* does not cause the breast tenderness, spotting or menstrual-type bleeding that are side effects of estrogen. In addition, *Evista®* did not increase the risk for breast cancer or cancer of the lining of the uterus in women studied for up to two and one-half years.

210

How do I use Evista®?

One *Evista®* tablet is taken once each day. This medication can be taken with or without food any time of the day. You must take *Evista®* as long as your doctor tells you to so that you can get the full benefit of the medication.

If you miss a dose of this medication, take it as soon as possible. However, if it is almost time for your next dose, skip the missed dose and go back to the dosing schedule. Do not double your dose. It is very important to take your medication exactly as directed by your doctor. NEVER stop taking your prescription medications without talking to your doctor.

In addition to *Evista®*, your doctor may recommend other important ways to prevent osteoporosis including weight-bearing exercise (such as walking), calcium, and vitamin D supplements, reducing use of alcohol (beer, wine, whiskey, etc.), and quitting smoking.

What side effects are possible from the use of Evista®?

The most common side effects are hot flashes (a sudden warm or hot feeling with sweating and reddening of the face and neck) and leg cramps.

A far less common, but much more serious side effect is blood clots of the veins, which can block the flow of blood and cause serious medical problems or even death. This is a problem that can also occur with estrogens. Call your doctor immediately if you have any of the following signs of blood clots:

• pain in the calves of the legs, or leg swelling (may mean there are blood clots in the legs)

• sudden chest pain or breathing problems, or coughing up blood (may mean there are blood clots in the lungs)

• changes in eyesight (may mean there are blood clots in the eyes)

Tell your doctor if you have side effects that do not go away over time, are bothersome, or stop you from taking your medication as directed.

Do other medications interact with Evista®?

If you are taking *Coumadin*® (warfarin) or other "blood thinners," your doctor may need to check your prothrombin time or INR (blood tests that measure how long it takes your blood to clot) when you first start taking *Evista*®. This test will tell whether or not your medication dose needs to be changed.

What else should I know about Evista®?

Be sure to tell your doctor if you have swelling of the hands, feet, or legs, bleeding from the vagina, breast pain, or an increase in the size of the breast while taking *Evista*®.

 ## Warning

You should not take *Evista*® if:

• You have or have had blood clots (including clots in the legs, lungs, or eyes) that needed treatment by a doctor.

• You have liver disease, unless your doctor recommends taking *Evista*®.

Calcium

Calcium is a mineral. It is an essential part of bones and is most important to the proper function of bodily organs. Most calcium in the body (99%) is located in bones. When the amount of calcium is decreased in the body, the body will "steal" calcium from bones. Therefore, it is important to keep giving the right amount of calcium to the body.

Most women in the United States don't get enough calcium in their diets. There are many different calcium supplement products, all of which work well. Calcium carbonate may cause gas. Some forms of calcium are combined with vitamin D. Avoid bone meal preparations because they may not be pure. Calcium will help slow bone loss in older women. It will <u>not</u> strengthen and thicken bones that have already been weakened by osteoporosis. Calcium alone will <u>not</u> prevent bone loss in early post-menopausal women. Calcium carbonate and calcium citrate are the most commonly used forms of calcium supplement.

Brand Name	Generic
Alka-Mints® Calcet® Plus Calcium Rich Rolaids® Caltrate® Os-Cal®	calcium carbonate
Calcium Lactate®	calcium lactate
Citracal®	calcium citrate
Neo-Calglucon® (syrup)	calcium glubionate calcium gluconate
Posture®	tribasic calcium phosphate

How do I use calcium?

Depending on how much supplement you need and the amount of elemental calcium in your tablets, you may have to take one to two tablets two to four times daily. Ask your doctor or pharmacist how to take it. Do not take calcium at the same time as other medications. Take it at least two hours apart from other medications.

If you miss a dose of this medication, take it as soon as possible. However, if it is almost time for your next dose, skip the missed dose and go back to the dosing schedule. Do not double your dose. It is very important to take your medication exactly as directed by your doctor. NEVER stop taking your prescription medications without talking to your doctor.

What side effects are possible from the use of calcium?

More Common

- constipation
- gas

Rare

Hypercalcemia (too much calcium) may occur with prolonged intake of high doses of calcium, especially when combined with vitamin D. This may cause:

- severe constipation
- stomach pain
- nausea, vomiting
- kidney stones
- great thirst
- weakness
- nervousness
- confusion

Tell your doctor if you have side effects that do not go away over time, are bothersome, or stop you from taking your medication as directed.

What else should I know about calcium?

• Remember to include a regular program of weight-bearing exercise, such as walking, gardening, etc., to prevent osteoporosis.

• Do not take antacids at the same time that you take calcium because antacids bind to calcium and won't allow calcium to be absorbed into the blood.

• Wait at least two hours before taking other medications.

• Men and women over 65 years old should have at least 1500 mg of elemental calcium daily. This may be obtained from calcium in your diet or from calcium supplements. Talk to your doctor or pharmacist for advice on calcium supplements.

• To absorb calcium, you need vitamin D. Some people do not get enough vitamin D in their diet. Talk to your doctor or pharmacist to see if you need to take a vitamin D supplement or multivitamin.

• Most calcium supplements are absorbed best when taken with food.

Recommended calcium intake (elemental calcium)

	Under 65	Over 65
Men	1000 mg	1500 mg
Pre-menopausal women	1000 mg	
Post-menopausal women +ERT*	1000 mg	1500 mg
Post-menopausal women -ERT*	1500 mg	1500 mg
* ERT = Estrogen Replacement Therapy		

Vitamin D

Vitamin D, made more active when your body gets sunlight, helps the body to absorb calcium. People require 400 IU of vitamin D daily which can be obtained from diet (milk and dairy products) or vitamin supplements. Older people, especially those who live in northern climates or who stay inside all day, may not get enough sunlight. These individuals can take a multivitamin that contains 400 IU of vitamin D.

Brand Name	Generic
Calderol®	calcifediol
DHT®, *Hytakerol*®	dihydrotachysterol
Rocaltrol®	calcitriol cholecalciferol

How do I use vitamin D?

Vitamin D also can be taken in combination with calcium. It is taken from once a day to once a week. 400 IU daily is required and can be obtained through dietary sources such as milk and dairy products or in a multivitamin. Several forms of vitamin D are available, some combined with calcium (*Os-Cal*® +D).

If you miss a dose, don't be concerned. Take your next scheduled dose as needed. Do not double your dose.

What side effects are possible from the use of vitamin D?

Less Common

If excess amounts are taken, they may produce hypercalcemia (too much calcium) leading to:

- severe constipation
- stomach pain
- nausea, vomiting
- kidney stones
- great thirst
- weakness
- nervousness
- confusion

Do other medications interact with vitamin D?

- The absorption of vitamin D into the blood is slowed down by mineral oil and *Questran®* (cholestyramine).

- Hypercalcemia (too much calcium) may cause irregular heartbeats (arrhythmia) in people taking *Lanoxicaps®* (digoxin) or *Calan®* (verapamil).

What else should I know about vitamin D?

- People taking corticosteroids or seizure medications, or people with chronic kidney failure, may need to take a vitamin D supplement or a multivitamin.

- Men and women over 65 years of age should have at least 1500 mg of elemental calcium daily. This may be obtained from calcium in your diet or from calcium supplements. Talk to your doctor or pharmacist for advice on calcium supplements.

 # Warning

- You do not need to take a vitamin D supplement with your calcium or with a multivitamin unless directed by your doctor.

Other agents

Bisphosphonates

Bisphosphonates prevent the release of calcium from bones.

Brand Name	Generic
Didronel®	etidronate
Fosamax®	alendronate

How do I use bisphosphonates?

Didronel® (etidronate) should be taken once daily. If stomach upset occurs it can be taken twice daily. It should be taken two hours apart from dairy products (milk, cheese, etc.), vitamins, and antacids. It is usually only taken for three months at a time.

Fosamax® (alendronate) is taken by mouth once a day. You should take Fosamax® first thing in the morning, at least 30 minutes before eating or drinking or taking any other medications. Take with a full glass (8 oz.) of water only. Do not lie down for at least 30 minutes after taking to prevent inflammation of the food pipe.

What side effects are possible from the use of bisphosphonates?

More Common

- headache
- gas
- acid backwash
- pain
- burning in the esophagus

Less Common

- rash
- fever
- bone pain
- low magnesium levels

Tell your doctor if you have side effects that do not go away over time, are bothersome, or stop you from taking your medication as directed.

Do other medications interact with bisphosphonates?

- Calcium and antacids slow down the absorption of bisphosphonates.

- Aspirin can <u>increase</u> stomach upset from *Fosamax®*.

- All medications <u>decrease</u> the absorption of *Fosamax®*.

What else should I know about bisphosphonates?

- Men and women over 65 years of age should have at least 1500 mg of elemental calcium daily. You can get this from calcium in your diet or from calcium supplements. Talk to your doctor or pharmacist for advice on calcium supplements.

• To absorb calcium you need vitamin D. Some people do not get enough vitamin D from their diet. Talk to your doctor or pharmacist to see if you need to take a vitamin D supplement or multivitamin.

Calcitonin

This medication is used to treat osteoporosis. It works in a similar way to *Fosamax®*. It prevents the release of calcium from bones. It can be given by injection or nasal spray.

Brand Name	Generic
Miacalcin®	calcitonin-salmon

How do I use calcitonin?

Calcitonin injection is given once a day. The nasal spray is given in one nostril every day, changing between nostrils each day. The nasal pump must be activated before the first use. Press down on the white side arms about six times until a faint spray comes out. There is no need to do this to the pump every day.

If you miss a dose, don't be concerned. Take your next scheduled dose as needed. Do not double your dose.

What side effects are possible from the use of calcitonin?

More Common

• nausea
• diarrhea
• facial flushing

- poor appetite
- headache
- runny nose (with nasal spray)

Less Common

- constipation
- rash
- itching
- swelling of feet

Tell your doctor if you have side effects that do not go away over time, are bothersome, or stop you from taking your medication as directed.

What else should I know about calcitonin?

- Unopened nasal spray should be stored in the refrigerator; once opened it may be stored at room temperature for up to one month.

- Men and women over 65 years of age should have at least 1500 mg of elemental calcium daily. This may be obtained from calcium in your diet or from calcium supplements. Talk to your doctor or pharmacist for advice on calcium supplements.

- To absorb calcium you need vitamin D. Some people do not get enough vitamin D from their diet. Talk to your doctor or pharmacist to see if you need to take a vitamin D supplement or a multivitamin.

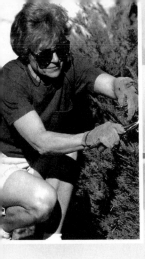

Parkinson's Disease

What is Parkinson's disease?

Parkinson's disease affects the way the nervous system controls the muscles in your body. When you move a part of your body, your brain sends messages through the body. The brain's signals are helped along by a chemical called dopamine. When you have Parkinson's disease, you don't have enough dopamine. This means that you will have problems with movement.

Symptoms may not be noticed at first, but get worse over time. The first signs are often shaking of the hand. Other symptoms include slowing or difficulty in movement, stiffness of muscles, and a shuffling walk. In later stages confusion, memory loss, and problems recognizing people and places may occur. Treatment with medication for Parkinson's is given to improve movement.

Medications used to treat Parkinson's disease

Anticholinergic Agents

Anticholinergic agents are most useful in younger patients, especially those with noticeable tremor and stiffness. Older people are more sensitive to this type of medication, making it less useful for them.

Brand Name	Generic
Akineton®	biperiden
Artane®	trihexyphenidyl
Benadryl®	diphenhydramine
Cogentin®	benztropine
Kemadrin®	procyclidine
Parsidol®	ethopropazine

How do I use anticholinergic agents?

Anticholinergic agents should be started at low dosages. They may be the first therapy used or added to other treatments for Parkinson's, such as Sinemet® (levodopa). Anticholinergic agents are taken one to several times a day. They should be taken with food to lessen the chance of an upset stomach.

If you miss a dose of this medication, take it as soon as possible. However, if it is almost time for your next dose, skip the missed dose and go back to the dosing schedule. Do not double your dose. It is very important to take your medication exactly as directed by your doctor. NEVER stop taking your prescription medications without talking with your doctor.

What side effects are possible from the use of anticholinergic agents?

More Common

- dry mouth
- blurred vision
- rapid heart beat

- widened pupils of the eye
- constipation
- problems emptying urine from the bladder

Less Common

- confusion
- skin flushing
- restlessness, irritability
- fever
- difficulty swallowing
- rash
- hallucinations (seeing strange, unreal visions)
- nausea
- light-headedness
- vomiting

Do other medications interact with anticholinergic agents?

Anticholinergics may _decrease_ the effects of:
- *Sinemet®* (levodopa)

Anticholinergics may _increase_ the effects of:
- narcotics
- antipsychotics
- antihistamines
- cyclic antidepressants

What else can anticholinergic agents be used for?

These medications are often used to treat the Parkinsonian-like side effects that occur with the use of some antipsychotic medications (used to treat certain mental conditions) or medications to prevent nausea.

What else should I know about anticholinergic agents?

Anticholinergic agents do not work for everyone. Talk to your doctor if your symptoms do not improve. You may be able to take something that will work better for you.

Sinemet® (Levodopa), known as L-Dopa

Sinemet® is a medication similar to a chemical found in the brain called dopamine. *Sinemet®* enters the brain and is converted to dopamine. It relieves the symptoms of Parkinson's disease. However, it does not stop the disease from getting worse. Unfortunately, *Sinemet®* becomes less effective over time.

Brand Name	Generic
Sinemet®, *Sinemet® CR*	levodopa/carbidopa

How do I use Sinemet®?

The stomach upset that often comes when first taking *Sinemet®* can be lessened by taking the medication with food. If the effects of the medication start to wear off before the next dose, it may be necessary to take the medication more often. Most people take it three times a day. Many of the side effects of *Sinemet®* are related to dose, which can be adjusted by your doctor. The controlled-release form of *Sinemet® CR* may be given in whole or half tablets but should not be crushed or chewed.

If you miss a dose of this medication, take it as soon as possible. However, if it is almost time for your next dose, skip the missed dose and go back to the dosing schedule. Do not double your dose. It is very important to take your medication exactly as directed by your doctor. NEVER stop taking your prescription medications without talking with your doctor.

What side effects are possible from the use of Sinemet®?

More Common

- confusion
- constipation
- nausea or vomiting
- uncontrollable movements
- light-headedness upon standing
- restlessness
- anxiety
- insomnia (trouble sleeping)
- nightmares
- difficulty urinating
- mood changes
- heart palpitations (a feeling of fast or pounding heartbeat in the chest)

Less Common

- flushing of the skin
- headache
- anorexia (decreased appetite)
- diarrhea
- eyelid twitching
- dry mouth

Tell your doctor if you have side effects that do not go away over time, are bothersome, or stop you from taking your medication as directed.

Do other medications interact with Sinemet®?

The following may *decrease* the effects of *Sinemet®*:
- Antipsychotics
- *Dilantin®* (phenytoin)
- *Reglan®* (metoclopramide)
- Vitamin B$_6$ (pyridoxine).
- *Parnate®* and *Nardil®* (non-selective monoamine oxidase inhibitors) may cause serious increases in blood pressure.

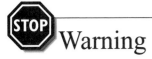 Warning

- Do not stop this medication suddenly, unless your doctor tells you to do so.

- Use carefully if you have glaucoma, an unidentified growth on the skin, or a history of melanomas (a form of skin cancer).

- Protein in the diet should be equally divided throughout the day to avoid fluctuations in the effects of *Sinemet®*.

Direct-Acting Dopamine Agonists

Dopamine agonists are medications which act at the same place on the brain as dopamine. They may help increase the effects of therapy with *Sinemet®*, particularly later in the disease.

Brand Name	Generic
Parlodel®	bromocriptine
Permax®	pergolide
Mirapex®	pramipexole

How do I use direct-acting dopamine agonists?

These medications are started in low doses and increased slowly until the right dose is found for you. *Parlodel®* (bromocriptine) and *Permax®* (pergolide) should be taken with food. *Mirapex®* (pramipexole) may be taken with food to ease the stomach upset that it can cause.

If you miss a dose of this medication, take it as soon as possible. However, if it is almost time for your next dose, skip the missed dose and go back to the dosing schedule. Do not double your dose. It is very important to take your medication exactly as directed by your doctor. NEVER stop taking your prescription medications without talking with your doctor.

What side effects are possible from the use of direct-acting dopamine agonists?

More Common

- dizziness
- nausea
- constipation
- insomnia (trouble sleeping)
- hallucinations (seeing strange, unreal visions)
- daytime sleepiness
- uncontrolled movements

Less Common

- memory problems
- loss of appetite
- dry mouth
- insomnia
- vomiting
- diarrhea
- shortness of breath
- swelling of hands and feet
- light-headedness upon standing

Rare

- blood disorders (low number of red or white blood cells)

Tell your doctor if you have side effects that do not go away over time, are bothersome, or stop you from taking your medication as directed.

Do other medications interact with direct-acting dopamine agonists?

- Antipsychotics (used to treat serious mental diseases) and *Reglan®* (metoclopramide) may <u>decrease</u> the effects of dopamine agonists.

- Erythromycin may <u>increase</u> the effects of *Parlodel®* (bromocriptine).

- *Tagamet®* (cimetidine), *Zantac®* (ranitidine), *Cardizem®* and *Cardizem® CD* (diltiazem), *Isoptin®*, *Isoptin® SR*, *Calan®* and *Calan® SR* (all brand names of verapamil), and *Quinaglute Dura-Tabs®*, *Quinidex Extentabs®* and *Cardioquin®* (all brand names of quinidine) may decrease the effect of *Mirapex®* (pramipexole).

What else should I know about direct-acting dopamine agonists?

- Usually the dose of *Sinemet®* is lowered after the desired dosage of the dopamine agonist is reached.

Indirect-Acting Dopamine Agonists

Indirect-acting dopamine agonists include *Eldepryl®* (selegiline), *Symadine®* and *Symmetrel®* (both brand names of amantadine). *Eldepryl®* is among the newest of the anti-Parkinsonian medications. It works by keeping more active dopamine in the brain. *Eldepryl®* is most commonly used with *Sinemet®* when there is a "wearing-off" effect of *Sinemet®*. It may also be used as the first therapy. That is because it may delay the time before *Sinemet®* is required.

The virus-fighting medications *Symadine®* and *Symmetrel®* are especially useful in the treatment of the flu among the elderly. In Parkinson's disease, *Symadine®* and *Symmetrel®* work by increasing the release of dopamine in the brain. *Symadine®* and *Symmetrel®* are not as effective as *Sinemet®* in controlling the shaking associated with Parkinson's disease, but it may work well for the stiffness.

Brand Name	Generic
Symmetrel®	amantadine
Symadine®	amantadine
Eldepryl®	selegiline

How do I use indirect-acting dopamine agonists?

Symadine®, *Symmetrel®* and *Eldepryl®* are taken by mouth, generally once or twice a day. Amantadine is available in syrup form.

If *Eldepryl®* is taken twice daily, it should be taken at breakfast and lunch to avoid trouble getting to sleep.

If you miss a dose of this medication, take it as soon as possible. However, if it is almost time for your next dose, skip the missed dose and go back to the dosing schedule. Do not double your dose. It is very important to take your medication exactly as directed by your doctor. NEVER stop taking your prescription medications without talking with your doctor.

What side effects are possible from the use of indirect-acting dopamine agonists?

More Common

- nausea, stomach pain
- dry mouth
- dizziness
- swelling of feet
- seizures
- confusion
- mood changes
- abnormal movements

Less Common

- fainting
- depression
- paranoia (unusual fears)
- insomnia (trouble sleeping)
- irritability
- blotchy rash
- light-headedness upon standing

Do other medications interact with indirect-acting dopamine agonists?

- Avoid using narcotics (codeine, morphine) and *Prozac*® (fluoxetine) at the same time as *Eldepryl*®.

- *Symadine*® and *Symmetrel*® _increase_ the side effects of anticholinergic medication; therefore, a lower dose may be needed.

- Hydrochlorthiazide and triamterene _increase_ the level of *Symadine*® and *Symmetrel*®.

What else can indirect-acting dopamine agonists be used for?

- *Symmetrel*® can be used for the flu and other viral infections.

- *Eldepryl*® has been used for Alzheimer's disease.

Warning

- *Eldepryl®* may cause a serious increase in blood pressure, especially if doses exceed 10 mg daily. If you are taking more than 10 mg a day, you will need to get a special diet from your doctor to prevent serious problems.

- Use *Symadine®* and *Symmetrel®* cautiously if you have a history of seizures, unexplained rashes, or liver disease.

Notes

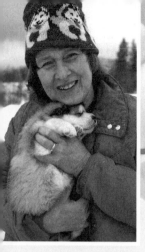

Sleep Problems and Nervousness

What are sleep problems (insomnia) and nervousness (anxiety)?

Insomnia (sleep problems)

Many people find that as they get older, they need less sleep and spend less time sleeping deeply at night. Although aging does affect sleep patterns, it is not "normal" for older people to <u>always</u> have problems getting a restful, good-night's sleep. Many older people complain of insomnia. Insomnia means taking a long time to fall asleep (more than 30 to 45 minutes), waking up many times at night, or waking up early and not being able to go back to sleep and not feeling rested in the morning.

Often, insomnia is caused by another problem. If you're having trouble sleeping you should talk with your doctor, who may recommend:

• Making it your routine to go to sleep and wake up at the same time every day.

• Getting moderate exercise every day. Don't exercise within two to four hours before bedtime.

• Avoiding caffeinated beverages (such as coffee, tea, cola) in the afternoon and avoiding alcoholic beverages (such as beer, wine, whiskey, etc.) altogether.

• Learning not to worry when you can't fall asleep.

• Taking medications that your doctor recommends.

Anxiety

Everyone has anxiety at one time or another. Anxiety is a feeling of fear, nervousness, tension, or stress. People suffering from anxiety may also feel other effects, such as increased heart rate and breathing, dizziness, headaches, muscle aches and pains, tiredness, shaking, or even chest and stomach pain. These symptoms can come and go as well.

Some anxiety is a natural response to danger or to dealing with difficult problems. But it's possible for anxiety to get in the way of everyday life. People who are anxious may shake, feel unsteady on their feet, and have a lot of fear. They may be cranky and have trouble sleeping and thinking clearly. Some people with anxiety may also feel depression, which is a feeling of sadness that doesn't go away.

Anxiety can be treated in many ways. Getting help from families or friends, talking with a doctor or counselor, or taking medications can lessen anxiety.

Medications used to treat sleep problems and anxiety

Benzodiazepines

Some benzodiazepines are best used for anxiety, while others should be used only for helping to get to sleep. The long-acting medications such as *Libritabs*® (chlordiazepoxide), *Librium*® (chlordiazepoxide), *Valium*® (diazepam), *Valrelease*® (diazepam), and *Dalmane*® (flurazepam) are less safe in older people because they stay in the body a very long time and are more likely to cause side effects (drowsiness), which may lead to falls, broken bones, and car accidents.

Benzodiazepines decrease anxiety and cause drowsiness.

"▲" Indicates medications that are <u>generally not recommended</u> for use in older people. Do not stop taking these medications unless directed by your doctor. They may be required under special circumstances. Talk to your doctor to see if this medication is right for you.

Brand Name	Generic
▲ *Centrax*®	prazepam
▲ *Dalmane*®	flurazepam
▲ *Doral*®	quazepam
▲ *Halcion*®	triazolam
▲ *Librax*®	chlordiazepoxide/clinidium
▲ *Libritabs*®	chlordiazepoxide
▲ *Librium*®	chlordiazepoxide
▲ *Paxipam*®	halazepam
▲ *Tranxene*®	clorazepate
▲ *Valium*®	diazepam
▲ *Valrelease*®	diazepam
▲ *Xanax*®	alprazolam
Ativan®	lorazepam
Klonopin®	clonazepam
ProSom®	estazolam
Restoril®	temazepam
Serax®	oxazepam

When needed for *anxiety*, the best choices of benzodiazepines for older persons are:

Ativan® (lorazepam) and *Serax*® (oxazepam).

When needed for *sleep*, the best choices of medications for older persons are:

Ambien® (zolpidem) and *Restoril*® (temazepam).

How do I use benzodiazepines?

For sleep, benzodiazepines are usually taken once before bedtime. For anxiety, they may be taken one to three times per day.

If you miss a dose, don't be concerned. Take your next scheduled dose as needed. Do not double your dose.

What side effects are possible from the use of benzodiazepines?

- agitation (feeling "hyper" or jittery)
- low blood pressure
- unsteady walking
- dizziness
- memory loss (especially for events that took place while using the medication)
- blurred (or double) vision
- slowed breathing (especially in people with lung disease)
- confusion
- urinary incontinence (no control of urine flow)
- daytime sleepiness
- grogginess
- colorful dreams

Tell your doctor if you have side effects that do not go away over time, are bothersome, or stop you from taking your medication as directed.

Do other medications interact with benzodiazepines?

The following medications, when taken in combination with benzodiazepines, *may result in increased drowsiness:*

- cold and allergy medications
- antidepressants
- narcotics
- antihistamines
- other antianxiety medications
- antipsychotics
- over-the-counter sleep medications
- *Tagamet*® (cimetidine)
- *Lopressor*® (metoprolol)
- *Prozac*® (fluoxetine)
- *Inderal*® (propanolol)
- *Nizoral*® (ketoconazole)
- *Depakene*® (valproic acid)
- alcohol (beer, wine, whiskey, etc.)

What else can benzodiazepines be used for?

People having problems trying to stop drinking alcohol (beer, wine, whiskey, etc.) may be treated with *Libritabs*®, *Librium*® (both chlordiazepoxide), *Valium*®, *Valrelease*® (both diazepam), or *Ativan*® (lorazepam). Seizure disorders, such as epilepsy, may be treated with *Klonopin*® (clonazepam), *Tranxene*® (clorazepate), *Valium*®, *Valrelease*®, or *Ativan*®.

What else should I know about benzodiazepines?

- Try to go to sleep without any medication first.

- If within 30 minutes you cannot fall asleep, take your sleep medication.

- Try breathing and relaxation exercises.

- Benzodiazepines cause drowsiness. Avoid activities requiring mental alertness such as driving a car, using sharp kitchen knives, or operating machinery.

- Do not drive or use alcohol (beer, wine, whiskey, etc.) when taking these medications.

- Take these medications for a short (three weeks or less) period of time; then talk with your doctor to decide if you need to continue taking the medication.

- Try not to use these medications every night.

 # Warning

- Benzodiazepines have a high risk for abuse (addiction) and dependence (feeling like you can't stop taking the medication).

- All medications that cause drowsiness are more likely to cause side effects in older people.

- Avoid long-acting benzodiazepines (refer to listing at beginning of section). They have too many side effects in older people.

- If you have liver disease, avoid all benzodiazepines, unless directed by your doctor.

- Never take more than the prescribed dose.

- DO NOT stop these medications abruptly if you have used them for a long time, unless told to do so by your doctor. Your doctor will instruct you on how to stop taking this medication if it is time. You should slowly cut down on your dose before stopping altogether.

- Since these medications may make you unsteady on your feet, you may be at risk for a fall which can lead to a broken bone. If you have a history of falling, be sure to tell your doctor. Your doctor may be able to change your medication to reduce your risk of falling.

Antihistamines

Antihistamines are not the best medications for the treatment of insomnia or anxiety, because they have a number of severe side effects in older people. They were developed to relieve allergy symptoms (sneezing, runny nose, itchy eyes, etc.). Yet, they also make people sleepy and are often used as sleep aids. These medications are found in many over-the-counter (OTC) sleeping pills and cold remedies.

"▲" Indicates medications that are <u>generally not recommended</u> for use in
older people. Do not stop taking these medications unless directed
by your doctor. They may be required under special circumstances.
Talk to your doctor to see if this medication is right for you.

Brand Name	Generic
▲ Atarax®	hydroxyzine
▲ Benadryl®	diphenhydramine
▲ Excedrin P.M.®	diphenhydramine
▲ Nytol® Maximum Strength	diphenhydramine
▲ Nytol® with DPH	diphenhydramine
▲ Sleep-Eze 3®	diphenhydramine
▲ Sominex® Formula 2	diphenhydramine
▲ Tylenol® P.M.	diphenhydramine
▲ Unisom® Nighttime Sleep Aid	doxylamine
▲ Vistaril®	hydroxyzine

How do I use antihistamines?

For sleep, these medications are generally taken once before bedtime.
For anxiety, they may be taken one to three times a day.

*If you miss a dose, don't be concerned. Take your next scheduled dose as
needed. Do not double your dose.*

What side effects are possible from the use of antihistamines?

- flushing (redness in the face)
- blurred vision
- dry mouth, nose, and throat
- memory problems
- confusion
- increased heartbeat
- constipation
- fainting
- diarrhea
- loss of appetite
- dizziness
- nausea and vomiting
- difficulty in urinating, especially in men with enlarged prostates (BPH)
- slowing of the reflexes

Tell your doctor if you have side effects that do not go away over time, are bothersome, or stop you from taking your medication as directed.

Do other medications interact with antihistamines?

The side effects may be made worse when antihistamines are taken with alcohol (beer, wine, whiskey, etc.), other antihistamines, or any other medications that cause drowsiness.

What else can antihistamines be used for?

Antihistamines can be used for allergic reactions, such as skin allergies or hay fever, or they can be used to dry up a runny nose due to the common cold.

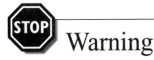 # Warning

Antihistamines are not generally recommended for use by older people for the treatment of anxiety or insomnia.

- Never take these medications in combination with alcoholic beverages (beer, wine, whiskey, etc.).

- Do not drive or perform other tasks that require mental alertness or quick reaction time.

- Antihistamines cause special problems for men with enlarged prostates or anyone with glaucoma.

- Although you can buy these medications over-the-counter, they are not good choices for anxiety or insomnia.

- Talk to your doctor if you have frequent insomnia or anxiety. Your doctor may be able to treat what is causing your symptoms or prescribe a medication for your symptoms.

- Never take more than the prescribed dose.

Noctec® (Chloral Hydrate)

Noctec® is used as a sleeping aid.

How do I use Noctec®?

Noctec® should be taken at bedtime. It is available in capsules, syrup, or suppository form.

If you miss a dose, don't be concerned. Take your next scheduled dose as needed. Do not double your dose.

What side effects are possible from the use of Noctec®?

More Common

- stomach pain, nausea/vomiting
- bad breath

Less Common

- excitement, light-headedness
- daytime drowsiness

Tell your doctor if you have side effects that do not go away over time, are bothersome, or stop you from taking your medication as directed.

Do other medications interact with Noctec®?

Noctec® may _increase_ the action of *Coumadin®* (warfarin), a blood thinner used to prevent or treat blood clots. It may also _increase_ the effect of alcohol (beer, wine, whiskey, etc.) and other medications that cause drowsiness.

What else should I know about Noctec®?

Avoid if you have liver or kidney failure, severe heart disease, or stomach problems.

 # Warning

- Never take more than the recommended dose.

- *Noctec®* may cause addiction if taken for a long period of time.

Buspar® (Buspirone)

This newer medication for the treatment of anxiety causes less drowsiness than most other medications.

How do I use Buspar®?

Buspar® is usually taken three times a day. Unlike other medications for anxiety, this medication takes several days to a week to become effective.

If you miss a dose, don't be concerned. Take your next scheduled dose as needed. Do not double your dose.

What side effects are possible from the use of Buspar®?

More Common

- dizziness
- nausea

Less Common

- restlessness
- excitement
- weakness
- headache

Tell your doctor if you have side effects that do not go away over time, are bothersome, or stop you from taking your medication as directed

Do other medications interact with Buspar®?

- Avoid taking other antianxiety, antidepressant, or antipsychotic agents while taking *Buspar®*.

- Do not take *Parnate®* and *Nardil®* (MAO inhibitors) when on *Buspar®*. Doing so may cause sudden, dangerous rises in blood pressure.

Ambien® (Zolpidem)

Ambien® is a newer type of sleep medication that works very quickly. As a result, you should only take this medication right before you go to bed and want to fall asleep.

The most common side effects reported in older people taking *Ambien®* were dizziness, drowsiness, and diarrhea. There is also the possibility that the medication can cause changes in the way you think and act. Because older people can be more sensitive to the effects of *Ambien®*, a low starting dose of 5 mg at bedtime is given to reduce the chance of side effects.

What else should I know about Ambien®?

- Do not drink alcohol (beer, wine, whiskey, etc.) when taking *Ambien®* because alcohol can _increase_ side effects.

- Until you know if *Ambien®* will make you drowsy the day after using it, do not drive or perform other tasks that require mental alertness or quick reaction time.

Meprobamate

In the past, this medication was prescribed often for anxiety, but it can cause a lot of drowsiness as well as life-threatening blood conditions. It is also addictive. In general, it is not a good choice for older people.

"▲" Indicates medications that are generally not recommended for use in older people. Do not stop taking these medications unless directed by your doctor. They may be required under special circumstances. Talk to your doctor to see if this medication is right for you.

Brand Name	Generic
▲ *Equanil*®	meprobamate
▲ *Meprospan*®	meprobamate
▲ *Miltown*®	meprobamate
▲ *Trancot*®	meprobamate

Barbiturates

Barbiturates should not be used to treat anxiety and insomnia. They are generally long-acting and lead to drowsiness and sluggishness on the day after use. Barbiturates are also highly addictive and interact with many other medications. People who have used them for a long time cannot suddenly stop them without having uncomfortable symptoms. Barbiturates may be used for treating seizures.

"▲" Indicates medications that are <u>generally not recommended</u> for use in older people. Do not stop taking these medications unless directed by your doctor. They may be required under special circumstances. Talk to your doctor to see if this medication is right for you.

Other agents

Brand Name	Generic
▲ *Amytal®*	amobarbital
▲ *Butisol®*	butabarbital
▲ *Luminal®*	phenobarbital
▲ *Nembutal®*	pentobarbital
▲ *Seconal®*	secobarbital

 Warning

• DO NOT stop these medications abruptly if you have used them for a long time, unless told to do so by your doctor. Your doctor will instruct you on how to stop taking this medication if it is time. You should slowly cut down on your dose before stopping altogether.

Notes

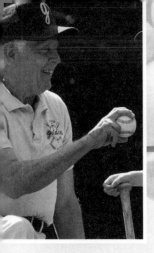

Stroke and Blood Clotting Prevention

What are stroke and blood clotting prevention agents (anticoagulant and antiplatelet agents)?

Blood clotting, a normal and desirable bodily process, occurs when proteins in the blood attach to platelets (tiny cells) to form a clot or plug. The process helps to stop bleeding following an injury.

Sometimes a clot forms in a blood vessel (thrombosis) which can block the normal flow of blood. A clot in one of the arteries that feeds the heart may result in a heart attack. A heart attack happens when part of the heart muscle dies because it doesn't get the oxygen that blood supplies. When a clot blocks one of the blood vessels of the brain, the affected part of the brain may die, which is called a stroke.

A clot in the veins of the leg, called a deep vein thrombosis, may occur following stomach or hip surgery or even after long periods of bed rest or a long plane or car ride. Such inactivity slows the flow of blood and lets it pool in the legs, increasing the chances of a clot forming. If such a clot breaks off, it may travel to the lungs, and a life-threatening disorder known as a pulmonary embolism may develop. Older adults are more at risk for abnormal clotting.

Medications that prevent the coagulation (clotting) of blood are called anticoagulants. Medications that prevent platelets (tiny blood cells that help start a clot) from sticking together to form clots are called antiplatelet medications and also help prevent clotting.

People who have had thrombosis or who have abnormal heart rhythms or valves are often given anticoagulation therapy. Anticoagulants cannot dissolve clots that have already formed, and do not actually "thin" the blood. They work by stopping clots from forming or existing clots from getting bigger, making it easier for the body to dissolve the clot.

Medications used to treat or prevent blood clotting

Anticoagulants

Anticoagulants decrease the production of proteins necessary for clotting so that it takes longer for a clot to form. Blood tests that measure how long blood takes to clot are used to adjust the dose of anticoagulant.

Older adults are sensitive to the effects of anticoagulants and must be watched very closely when using this medication.

Brand Name	Generic
Coumadin®	warfarin
Dicumarol®	dicumarol
Miradon®	anisindione

How do I use anticoagulants?

Anticoagulants are usually taken once a day. It is best to take anticoagulants on an empty stomach because they may interact with a number of foods or other medications. The dose is adjusted based on blood tests; never change your dose except on the advice of your doctor.

If you miss a dose of this medication, take it as soon as possible. However, if it is almost time for your next dose, skip the missed dose and go back to the dosing schedule. Do not double your dose. It is very important to take your medication exactly as directed by your doctor. NEVER stop taking your prescription medications without talking with your doctor.

What side effects are possible from the use of anticoagulants?

Less Common
- bleeding or hemorrhage
- bruising
- diarrhea
- nausea
- vomiting
- stomach cramps

Rare
- severe peeling skin rash
- hair loss
- dark urine
- inflammation of the liver
- jaundice (yellowing of skin and whites of eyes)
- skin sores

Tell your doctor if you have side effects that do not go away over time, are bothersome, or stop you from taking your medication as directed.

Do other medications interact with anticoagulants?

Because many medications interact with anticoagulants changes in dosage are sometimes necessary. <u>Drug interactions can be very severe.</u> Never start or stop any drug without asking your doctor.

Some of the commonly used medications that *increase* the anticoagulant action of anticoagulants include:

- *Anturane®* (sulfinpyrazone)

- *Aquachloral®* (chloral hydrate)

- *Atromid-S®* (clofibrate)

- *Bufferin®, Anacin®, Excedrin®* (aspirin)

- *Butazolidin®* (phenylbutazone)

- *Dilantin®* (phenytoin)

- *Ery-Tab®, PCE®* (erythromycin)

- *Flagyl®* (metronidazole)

- *Nizoral®* (ketoconazole)

- non-steroidal anti-inflammatory drugs (NSAIDs)

- oral hypoglycemics

- *Quinaglute®* (quinidine)

- *Synthroid®* (thyroid medications)

- *Tagamet®* (cimetidine)

- *Tylenol®* (acetaminophen)

Some of the medications that *decrease* the effects of warfarin derivatives are:

- barbiturates

- *Colestid®* (colestipol)

- *Questran®* (cholestyramine)

- *Rifadin®* (rifampin)

- *Tegretol®* (carbamazepine)

- vitamin K

What else should I know about anticoagulants?

- Wear a MedicAlert bracelet.

- Avoid vitamin K, which is found in green leafy vegetables, liver, and green tea. Do not take vitamin K preparations unless instructed to do so by a doctor. Do not make changes in your diet without talking to your doctor.

- Stomach pain may be the sign of an ulcer. If ulcers are left untreated, they may cause serious bleeding. Tell your doctor if you have stomach pain that is severe or keeps returning, or if you have a history of peptic ulcer disease. Call your doctor immediately if you notice dark, coffee-grounds looking stool, or if you are vomiting dark material that looks like coffee grounds. These may be signs of a bleeding ulcer.

- Never add or stop a prescription or over-the-counter medication without first talking with your doctor.

 ## Warning

- Jaundice (yellowing of the skin and/or whites of the eyes) may be a sign of liver damage and should be reported to your doctor as soon as possible.

- *Tylenol*® (acetaminophen) may increase the effects of *Coumadin*® (warfarin).

Heparin (heparin sodium)

When given either into the vein or under the skin, *Heparin* (heparin sodium) has powerful anticoagulant activities. *Heparin* cannot be taken by mouth.

Heparin is generally given when clot prevention must be started quickly. In the elderly it is sometimes given before and after surgery to prevent blood clots and pulmonary embolism.

Brand Name	Generic
Heparin Calciparine®	heparin sodium
Lovenox®	enoxaparin

How do I use Heparin?

Heparin is given intravenously (into the bloodstream) or by injection.

If given at home, it is usually twice daily, injected under the skin. Injections are usually given in the stomach area.

What side effects are possible from the use of Heparin?

More Common
- chills
- fever
- skin rash
- itching and burning of the feet

Less Common
- bleeding or hemorrhage (the main complication of treatment)
- skin irritation at the site of injection

Rare
- asthma
- rhinitis
- headache
- nausea
- vomiting

Tell your doctor if you have side effects that do not go away over time, are bothersome, or stop you from taking your medication as directed.

Do other medications interact with Heparin?

The following medications may _increase_ the risk of bleeding (hemorrhage) and should be used carefully in patients receiving _Heparin_.

- aspirin

- _Butazolidin_® (phenylbutazone)

- cephalosporin antibiotics

- _Coumadin_® (warfarin)

- _D.H.E. 45_® (dihydroergotamine)

- _Nitro-Dur_®, _Transderm-Nitro_® (nitrogylcerin)

- non-steroidal anti-inflammatory drugs (NSAIDs)

- penicillin antibiotics

- _Persantine_® (dipyridamole)

- _Plaquenil_® (hydroxychloroquine)

- _Ticlid_® (ticlopidine)

What else should I know about Heparin?

Heparin may also be used for prevention and treatment of venous thrombosis (clot formation in the veins), treatment of atrial fibrillation (rapid, irregular heartbeat), prophylaxis, and treatment of clots in the arteries.

 Warning

- You should not receive _Heparin_ if you have an uncontrolled bleeding disorder.

- _Heparin_ should be discontinued if a patient experiences nosebleeds, black, tarry stools, and/or blood in the urine.

• Stomach pain may be the sign of an ulcer. If ulcers are left untreated, they may cause serious bleeding. Tell your doctor if you have stomach pain that is severe or keeps returning, or if you have a history of peptic ulcer disease. Call your doctor immediately if you notice dark, coffee-grounds looking stool, or if you are vomiting dark material that looks like coffee grounds. These may be signs of a bleeding ulcer.

Aspirin

Because aspirin slows coagulation, it helps to prevent heart attacks and certain kinds of strokes.

Although aspirin is an inexpensive over-the-counter drug, it should not be taken on a daily basis except on the advice of your doctor.

Brand Name	Generic
Acuprin® Adult Low Dose Aspirin	aspirin
Bayer® Aspirin Maximum Strength	aspirin
Bayer® Aspirin (regular strength)	aspirin
Bayer® Children's Aspirin	aspirin
Bayer® Enteric-Coated	aspirin
Ecotrin®	aspirin
St. Josephs® Adult Aspirin	aspirin

How do I use aspirin?

A number of aspirin products are coated or have added ingredients called *buffers* to make the medication less damaging to the stomach. Buffers may reduce some, but not all, of the side effects. Do not crush or chew these pills. Take the medication with a full 8-ounce glass of water on a full stomach to prevent pills from sticking in your throat.

If you miss a dose, don't be concerned. Take your next scheduled dose as needed. Do not double your dose. It is very important to take your medication exactly as directed by your doctor. NEVER stop taking your prescription medications without talking with your doctor.

What side effects are possible from the use of aspirin?

More Common
- nausea or vomiting
- heartburn (dyspepsia)

Less Common
- ringing in the ears (tinnitus) or hearing loss
- stomach ulcers/bleeding
- iron-poor anemia
- bruising

Rare
- allergic reactions: skin rash, hives, itching, swelling of face and throat, shortness of breath
- severe bleeding
- salicylism: dizziness, diarrhea, confusion, headache, sweating, hyperventilation

Tell your doctor if you have side effects that do not go away over time, are bothersome, or stop you from taking your medication as directed.

Do other medications interact with aspirin?

Aspirin may *increase* the effects of the following medications:

- anticoagulants (blood thinners)

- *Depakote®, Depakene®* (valproic acid)

- *Rheumatrex®* (methotrexate)

Aspirin may _decrease_ the effects of the following medications:

- *Anturane*® (sulfinpyrazone)

- *Benemid*® (probenecid)

- blood pressure medications

- diuretics (water pills)

What else can aspirin be used for?

Aspirin is also used for pain, arthritis, and fever.

 # Warning

- It can be hard to know if you are taking too much aspirin; tinnitus (ringing in the ears) and hearing loss may be signs you are taking too much medication.

- Aspirin can decrease blood clotting. It has a long effect on platelets that help blood clot. It should be stopped one week prior to surgery.

- Do not take aspirin if you are taking blood thinners, such as warfarin, unless told to by your doctor.

- Aspirin should not be used by children (under 18 years of age) because it may cause Reye's syndrome, a life-threatening condition that can lead to coma and death. Keep this and all medications away from young children.

- Allergic reactions may produce a skin rash and wheezing with difficulty in breathing. Do not take aspirin if you have had a bad reaction to aspirin or any other non-steroidal anti-inflammatory medications (NSAIDs) in the past.

- Stomach pain may be a sign of an ulcer. If ulcers are left untreated, they may cause serious bleeding. Tell your doctor if you have stomach pain that is severe or keeps coming back or if you have a history of peptic ulcer disease. Call your doctor immediately if you notice dark, tarry-looking stools or if you are vomiting dark material that looks like coffee grounds. These may be signs of a bleeding ulcer.

- People with kidney disease, liver disease, or congestive heart failure may experience worsening of these illnesses. Be sure to tell your doctor if you have these conditions. If you have these conditions, talk to your doctor before taking any OTC medications, including aspirin and NSAIDs, which are available over the counter.

- Alcohol (beer, wine, whiskey, etc.) increases the chance of stomach ulceration and bleeding. Avoid alcohol (beer, wine, whiskey, etc.) or limit alcohol while taking aspirin.

- Do not take aspirin, or any other combination medication containing aspirin, unless instructed by your doctor.

- If your doctor does tell you to take aspirin, take only the amount of aspirin ordered by your doctor.

Notes

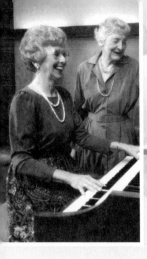

Underactive Thyroid

What is underactive thyroid (hypothyroidism)?

The thyroid is a small gland that sits at the base of the neck. It produces a hormone (a natural chemical) that controls many important jobs in the body. The thyroid helps to keep skin, hair, bones, and teeth healthy; controls body temperature and energy; and keeps you thinking clearly. When the thyroid does not produce enough thyroid hormone, it is underactive. This condition is called hypothyroidism.

Hypothyroidism is common in older people, especially women. Some older people have symptoms and others do not. If you have hypothyroidism, you may have one or more of the following symptoms:

• low tolerance to cold (not feeling well during cold weather)
• decreased appetite
• weight gain
• drowsiness
• dry skin
• shortness of breath
• slow speech
• depression (sadness that doesn't go away)
• nausea
• constipation
• edema (swelling from fluid buildup)

Hypothyroidism is most commonly treated with medications.

Medications used to treat underactive thyroid

Thyroid Medications

Thyroid hormone medications are taken to replace the thyroid hormone that the thyroid gland can no longer produce. They may also be used to keep a goiter (a bulging neck caused by an enlarged thyroid) from forming or growing. These medications are made in a laboratory or taken from animal sources. *Levothroid*® and *Synthroid*® (both brand names of levothyroxine) are synthetic preparations similar to the natural human hormone. *Armour*® *Thyroid*, *Thyrolar*® (both brand names of thyroid USP) and *Proloid*® (thyroglobulin) are prepared from the thyroid glands of animals but are rarely used these days. *Levothroid*® and *Synthroid*® are the best forms of therapy for most people because of their strength and reliability. They are man-made in a laboratory and are more reliable than thyroid hormones made from animal sources.

Brand Name	Generic
Armour® *Thyroid*	thyroid USP
Cytomel®	liothyronine
Euthroid®	liotrix
Levothroid®	levothyroxine
Proloid®	thyroglobulin
Synthroid®	levothyroxine
Thyrolar®	thyroid USP

How do I use thyroid medications?

Thyroid medication is generally taken once a day. The dose is started very low, especially in older people, and increased slowly. If the dose is started too high, you may have side effects. If the dose is too low, you may not get better. You should start to feel better in the first month, but it may take longer. Thyroid function tests are blood tests used to measure how much thyroid medication you need and how well it is working. Doses are often changed after the blood test results.

If you miss a dose of this medication, take it as soon as possible. However, if it is almost time for your next dose, skip the missed dose and go back to the dosing schedule. Do not double your dose. It is very important to take your medication exactly as directed by your doctor. NEVER stop taking your prescription medications without talking with your doctor.

What side effects are possible from the use of thyroid medications?

Since *Levothroid*® and *Synthroid*® are nearly identical to what is naturally produced by your body, they cause few side effects. Most side effects occur only when the dose is too high.

Symptoms of toxicity (too much thyroid medication):

- rapid heartbeat/chest pain
- sweating
- flushing of the skin
- confusion
- diarrhea
- not feeling well during hot weather
- weight loss
- shortness of breath
- insomnia (trouble sleeping)
- nervousness

Tell your doctor if you have side effects that do not go away over time, are bothersome, or stop you from taking your medication as directed.

Do other medications interact with thyroid medications?

- Thyroid hormones may *increase* the effects of *Coumadin*® (warfarin). Your doctor should check your bleeding carefully when starting, stopping, or changing the dose of thyroid medication. Tell your doctor if you notice any bruising or bleeding.

- *Questra*® (cholestyramine), *Colestid*® (colestipol used for high cholesterol) and iron supplements may lessen the amount of thyroid hormone taken in by the body. Take thyroid hormone two hours before or four hours after these medications.

- Thyroid hormone may change the amount of insulin or other diabetes medication needed. Blood sugar may change when starting or stopping thyroid medication. Your doctor may need to change your dose of insulin or oral diabetic medication.

- The dose of *Lanoxin*® and *Lanoxicaps*® (both are the brand names of digoxin) may need to be changed when thyroid medication is started, stopped, or the dose is changed.

- Over-the-counter (OTC) cough and cold medications can *increase* the side effects of thyroid medications. Ask your doctor or pharmacist before taking any OTC medications.

What else should I know about thyroid medications?

- People with a history of heart disease, angina (chest pain), or a past myocardial infarction (heart attack) must be especially careful when starting thyroid hormone medications. The beginning dose is usually low and increased slowly by your doctor to prevent side effects.

• Thyroid hormone affects the health of your bones. Too much thyroid hormone (too high of a dose) can make it more likely for you to get osteoporosis (brittle bones). Talk with your doctor about osteoporosis and ways that you can help prevent it.

• Always remember to tell your doctor about your history of thyroid disease and include thyroid hormone when asked to list your medications.

• When you first start thyroid medication, your doctor will check how well your thyroid is working every month or so until it is working steadily. After it is working steadily, your doctor should check your thyroid function about every 6 to 12 months.

 Warning

Do not stop or change the dose of your thyroid medication unless directed by your doctor.

Notes

GLOSSARY

"▲": Indicates medications that are generally not recommended for use in older people.

Absorption: The uptake of substances into or across tissues.

Acute: Short-lived and intense.

Addiction: A development of dependency on a medication.

Analgesic: Having the ability to stop pain.

Angina: Chest pain due to coronary artery disease.

Anxiety: A feeling of fear, nervousness, or tension.

Anticoagulant: A medication that prevents the blood from clotting.

Arrhythmia: Irregular heart pulse.

Artery: Any of the tubular branching vessels that carry blood from the heart through the body.

Arthritis: Inflammation of the joints.

Asthma: A disease of the lungs that causes episodes of wheezing, coughing, shortness of breath, and tightness in the chest.

Blood clots: A semisolid mass formed of blood, either in or out of the body.

Blood vessel: A special tube that carries blood throughout the body.

Chronic: Long-term.

Congestive Heart Failure: A condition in which the heart cannot pump enough blood to meet the body's needs.

Constipation: A condition in which there is a decreased number of bowel movements and the passing of hard stools.

Coronary Artery Disease: A disease in which the arteries that supply blood to the heart are narrowed by fatty deposits.

COPD (Chronic Obstructive Airway Disease): Including emphysema and chronic bronchitis, a type of disease in which the airways are blocked in the lungs.

Depression: A disorder marked by long-term sadness, inactivity, difficulty thinking and concentrating, and feelings of hopelessness.

Diabetes: A disease that lessens the body's ability to use food properly.

Diuretic: A type of medication that helps the kidneys get rid of water and salt from the body.

Drug interactions: Incidents that occur in the body when a medication is affected by another medication or food.

Estrogen: A hormone made by the ovaries in a woman's body.

Glaucoma: A disease in which there is too much fluid pressure in the eye.

Glucose: A sugar found in certain foods and in the normal blood of all animals that is the chief source of energy for living organisms.

Heart Failure: See "Congestive Heart Failure."

High Blood Pressure: A condition in which pressure of blood against the artery walls is consistently higher than normal.

Hyperglycemia: A condition in which there is too much glucose in the blood.

Hypertension: See "High Blood Pressure."

Hypoglycemia: A condition in which there is too little glucose in the blood.

Hypothyroidism: A condition in which not enough thyroid hormone is produced in the body.

Indigestion: Painful or difficult digestion.

Insomnia: Difficulty sleeping at night.

Irritable Bowel Syndrome: A condition in which an oversensitive gastrointestinal tract may result in constipation, diarrhea, pain, bloating, and cramping.

MedicAlert Bracelet: A special bracelet that states important medical information that is worn by people who have medical conditions. These medical bracelets can help medical personnel help the individual in case of emergency.

Nebulizer: A machine that helps to deliver inhaled medication.

Osteoporosis: The abnormal reduction of bone mass and strength.

OTC (over-the-counter): Any medication that can be bought without a prescription.

Pain: An unpleasant feeling or sensation.

Parkinson's disease: Disease that affects the way the nervous system controls the muscles in one's body.

Side effect: Any unwanted physical or mental state caused as a result of using a drug; also called "adverse effect."

Thrombosis: A condition in which a blood clot forms in a blood vessel.

Ulcer: Sores on the lining of the stomach or small intestine.

List of Brand Names and Manufacturers

Brand Name	Manufacturer
Accolate®	Zeneca
Accupril®	Parke-Davis
Achromycin®	Lederle
Acuprin®	Richwood
Adalat®	Bayer
Adrenalin®	Parke-Davis
Adsorbocarpine®	Alcon Opthalmics
Advil®	Whitehall
AeroBid®	Forest
Agoral®	Warner-Lambert Consumer
Akineton®	Knoll Labs
Alamag®	Goldline
Aldactazide®	Searle
Aldactone®	Searle
▲ Aldomet®	Merck
Aleve®	Procter & Gamble
Alka-Mints®	Bayer
Alka-Seltzer®	Miles
Alkets®	Roberts Pharmaceutical, Inc.
Alphagan®	Allergan
Altace®	Hoechst Marion Roussel
AlternaGEL®	J & J-Merck
Alupent®	Boehringer Ingelheim
Amaryl®	Hoechst Marion Roussel
Ambien®	Searle
Amitone®	Menley & James

Brand Name	Manufacturer
Amoxil®	SmithKline Beecham
Amphojel®	Wyeth-Ayerst
▲ Amytal®	Lilly
Anacin®	Whitehall, Roche, Wyeth-Ayerst
Anaprox®	Roche Laboratories
▲ Anaspaz®	Ascher
Ansaid®	Upjohn
Antabuse®	Wyeth-Ayerst
Anturane®	Novartis
Aquachloral®	Polymedica Pharmaceutical
Aristocort®	Fujisawa
Armour® Thyroid	Forest
Artane®	Lederle Labs
Arthritis Pain Formula®	Medtech Labs
Ascriptin®	Rhone-Poulenc Rorer
Asendin®	Lederle Labs
AsthmaHaler Mist®	Menley & James
AsthmaNefrin®	Menley & James
▲ Atarax®	Pfizer
Ativan®	Wyeth-Ayerst
Atromid-S®	Wyeth-Ayerst
▲ Atropine®	Arco
Atrovent®	Boehringer Ingelheim
Axid®	Lilly
Azmacort®	Rhone-Poulenc Rorer
Azulfidine®	Pharmacia & Upjohn

Brand Name	Manufacturer	Brand Name	Manufacturer
Bactrim®	Roche Laboratories	▲ Butisol®	Wallace
Basaljel®	Wyeth-Ayerst	Cafergot®	Sandoz
Bayer® Aspirin	Bayer	Calan®	Searle
Bayer Aspirin Maximum®	Bayer	Calcet Plus®	Mission
Bayer Children's Aspirin®	Bayer	Calcium Lactate®	Glenwood Palisades
Enteric-Coated Bayer®	Bayer	Calcium Rich Rolaids®	American Chicle
Beclovent®	Glaxo Wellcome	Calderol®	Organon
Bellafoline®	Sandoz	Caltrate®	Lederle
Bell/ans®	Dent, C.S.	▲ Cantil®	Hoechst Marion Roussel
▲ Benadryl®	Warner-Lambert Consumer	Capoten®	Bristol-Myers Squibb
Benemid®	Merck	Capozide®	Bristol-Myers Squibb
▲ Bentyl®	Hoechst Marion Roussel	Carafate®	Hoechst Marion Roussel
Betagan®	Allergan	Cardarone®	Wyeth-Ayerst
Betaloc®	Astra	Cardene®	Roche Laboratories
Betapace®	Berlex	Cardioquin®	Purdue Frederick
Betoptic®	Alcon Laboratories	Cardizem®	Hoechst Marion Roussel
Biaxin®	Abbott	Cartrol®	Abbott
Blocadren®	Merck	Catapres®	Boehringer Ingelheim
Brethaire®	Geigy	Celestone®	Schering
Brethine®	Novartis	▲ Centrax®	Parke-Davis
Bricanyl®	Hoechst Marion Roussel	Chlortrimeton®	Schering-Plough
Bronkaid Mist®	Sterling Health	Chooz®	Schering-Plough
Bronkometer®	Sanofi	Chronulac®	Marion Merrell Dow
Bronkosol®	Sanofi	Cipro®	Bayer
Bufferin®	Bristol-Myers Products	Citracal®	Mission
Bumex®	Roche Laboratories	Citrocarbonate®	Roberts
Buspar®	Bristol-Myers Squibb	Citrucel®	SmithKline Beecham
▲ Butazoldin®	Geigy	Climara®	Berlex Labs

Brand Name	Manufacturer	Brand Name	Manufacturer
Clinoril®	Merck	▲ Demerol®	Sanofi
Cogentin®	Merck	Depakene®	Abbott
Colace®	Roberts	Depakote®	Abbott
Colestid®	Pharmacia & Upjohn	Deponit®	Schwarz
Combivent®	Boehringer Ingelheim	Desyrel®	Apothecon
Compoz®	Medtech	Diabeta®	Hoechst Marion Roussel
Cordarone®	Wyeth-Ayerst	▲ Diabinese®	Pfizer
Corgard®	Bristol-Myers Squibb	Dialose®	J & J-Merck
Cortef®	Upjohn	Dialose Plus®	J & J-Merck
Cortone®	Merck	Diamarol®	Abbott
Coumadin®	Dupont	Diamox®	Lederle Labs
Creon 10®	Solvay	Dicarbosil®	SmithKline Beecham
▲ Cystospaz®	PolyMedica	Dicumarol®	Abbott
Cytomel®	SmithKline Beecham	Didronel®	Procter & Gamble
Cytotec®	Searle	Diflucan®	Pfizer
DHE 45®	Sandoz	Di-Gel®	Schering-Plough
DHT®	Roxane	Dilacor®	Rhone-Poulenc Rorer
▲ Dalmane®	Roche Products	Dilantin®	Parke-Davis
Daranide®	Merck	Dilatrate-SR®	Schwarz
▲ Darvocet-N®	Lilly	Dilaudid®	Knoll Labs
▲ Darvon®	Lilly	Disalcid®	3M
Darvon Compound-65®	Lilly	Dispos-a-Med®	Parke-Davis
Daypro®	Searle	Diucardin®	Wyeth-Ayerst
Decadron®	Merck	Diuril®	Merck
Decatron® Phospate	Merck	Dolobid®	Merck
Delta-Cortef®	Upjohn	▲ Donnatal®	Robins
Deltasone®	Upjohn	▲ Doral®	Wallace
Demadex®	Boehringer Mannheim	Dulcolax®	Novartis Consumer
		Duo-Medihaler®	3M

Brand Name	Manufacturer	Brand Name	Manufacturer
Duract®	Wyeth-Ayerst	▲ Excedrin PM®	Bristol-Myers
Dyazide®	SmithKline Beecham	Ex-Lax®	Sandoz
Dymelor®	Lilly	Feldene®	Pfizer
Dynacirc®	Novartis	FiberCon®	Lederle
Dyrenium®	SmithKline Beecham	Flagyl®	Searle
Ecotrin®	SmithKline Beecham Consumer	Fleet®	Fleet
		Fleet Phospho-Soda®	Fleet
Edecrin®	Merck	Floropryl®	Merck
Effexor®	Wyeth-Ayerst	Flovent®	Glaxo Wellcome
▲ Elavil®	Zeneca	Fosamax®	Merck
Eldepryl®	Somerset	Gaviscon®	SmithKline Beecham
Empirin®	Warner-Wellcome	Gelusil®	Warner Wellcome
E-Mycin®	Knoll	Glucophage®	Bristol-Myers Squibb
Enduron®	Abbott	Glucotrol®	Pfizer
Epifrin®	Allergan	Glynase®	Pharmacia & Upjohn
▲ Equanil®	Wyeth-Ayerst	▲ Halcion®	Pharmacia & Upjohn
Equilet®	Mission	Haldol®	Ortho-McNeil
Ergomar®	Lotus	Halfprin®	Kramer
Eryc®	Parke-Davis	Heparin®	Wyeth-Ayerst
Ery-Tab®	Abbott	Hexadrol®	Organon
Eskalith®	SmithKline Beecham	Humorsol®	Merck
Estrace®	Bristol-Meyers	Hydrocortone®	Merck
Estraderm®	Novartis	Hygroton®	Rhone-Poulenc Rorer
Estratabb®	Solvay	Imodium®	Janssen
Ethmozine®	Roberts	Inderal®	Wyeth-Ayerst
Euthroid®	Parke-Davis	Inderal LA®	Wyeth-Ayerst
Evista®	Eli-Lilly	Inderide®	Wyeth-Ayerst
Excedrin®	Bristol-Myers	▲ Indocin®	Merck

Brand Name	Manufacturer	Brand Name	Manufacturer
Intal®	Rhone-Poulenc Rorer	Lopid®	Parke-Davis
Ismelin®	Novartis	Lopressor®	Novartis
Isonate®	various	Lortab®	UCB
Isoptin®	Knoll Labs	Losopan®	Zenith/Goldline
Isopto Carbachol®	Alcon Opthalmics	Lotensin®	Novartis
Isopto Carpine®	Alcon Opthalmics	Lovenox®	Rhone-Poulenc Rorer
Isordil®	Wyeth-Ayerst	Lozol®	Rhone-Poulenc Rorer
Isosorbide®	Alcon Opthalmics	Ludiomil®	Ciba
Kaopectate®	Pharmacia & Upjohn	▲ Luminal®	Abbott Hospital Products Sanofi Winthrop
Kemadrin®	Glaxo Wellcome	MS Contin®	Purdue Frederick
Kerlone®	Searle	Maalox®	Novartis Consumer
Klonopin®	Roche Laboratories	Magan®	Savage
Kondremul®	Novartis	Magnalox®	Private label
Konsyl®	Konsyl	Mallamint®	Roberts
Kudrox®	Schwarz	Maltsupex®	Wallace
Lanoxicaps®	Glaxo Wellcome	Marblen®	Fleming
Lanoxin®	Glaxo Wellcome	Maxair®	3M
Lasix®	Hoechst Marion Roussel	Meclofenamate®	Mylan
Levato®	Schwarz	Meclomen®	Parke-Davis
Levothroid®	Forest	Medihaler-Iso®	3M
▲ Levsin®	Schwarz	Medrol®	Upjohn
▲ Librax®	Roche Products	Mellaril®	Sandoz Pharmaceuticals
▲ Libritabs®	Roche	Menest®	SmithKline Beecham
▲ Librium®	Roche Products	▲ Meprospan®	Wallace
Lithobid®	Solvay	Metamucil®	Procter & Gamble
Lithonate®	Solvay	Metaprel®	Sandoz
Lithotabs®	Solvay	Meticorten®	Schering
Lodine®	Wyeth-Ayerst		

Brand Name	Manufacturer	Brand Name	Manufacturer
Mexitil®	Boehringer Ingelheim	Nitro-Bid®	Hoechst Marion Roussel
Miacalcin®	Sandoz	Nitrocap TD®	North American
Micronase®	Pharmacia & Upjohn	Nitrodisc®	Roberts
Midamor®	Merck	Nitro-Dur®	Key
Milk of Magnesia®	Pharmaceutical Associates	Nitrogard®	Forest
▲ Miltown®	Wallace	Nitroglyn®	Kenwood
Minizide®	Pfizer	Nitrol®	Savage
Miradon®	Schering	Nitrolingual®	Rhone-Poulenc Rorer
Mirapex®	Pharmacia & Upjohn	Nitrospan®	Rhone-Poulenc Rorer
Mitrolan®	Robins	Nitrostat®	Parke-Davis
Mobidin®	Ascher	Nizoral®	Janssen
Moduretic®	Merck	Noctec®	Bristol-Myers Squibb
Monopril®	Bristol-Myers Squibb	Normodyne®	Schering
Motrin®	McNeil Consumer	▲ Norpace®	Searle
Mylanta®	J & J-Merck	Norpramin®	Hoechst Marion Roussel
Nalfon®	Dista	Norvasc®	Pfizer
Naprosyn®	Roche Laboratories	▲ Nytol®	Block
Nardil®	Parke-Davis	▲ Nytol ® with DPH	Block
Nature's Remedy®	SmithKline Beecham Consumer	Nytol® Max. Strength	Block
Navane®	Pfizer	Ogen®	Pharmacia & Upjohn
NebuPent®	Fujisama	Orap®	Gate
▲ Nembutal®	Abbott	Orasone®	Reid-Rowell
Neo-Calglucon®	Sandoz	Orinase®	Upjohn
Neoloid®	Kenwood Labs	Ortho-Est®	Ortho Pharmaceuticals
Neoral®	Sandoz	Orudis®	Wyeth-Ayerst
Neotabs®	Pharma-Tek	Oruvail®	Wyeth-Ayerst
Neptazane®	Lederle Labs	Os-Cal+D®	SmithKline Beecham Consumer
		PCE®	Abbott

Brand Name	Manufacturer
P.V. Carpine®	Allergan Switz
Pamelor®	Sandoz
Panadol®	SmithKline Beecham
Pancrease®	McNeil Pharmaceutical
Panex®	Roberts
Parlodel®	Novartis
Parnate®	SmithKline Beecham
Parsidol®	Parke-Davis
Paxil®	SmithKline Beecham
▲ Paxipam®	Schering
Pentam®	Fujisama
Penvee K®	Wyeth-Ayerst
Pepcid®	Merck
Pepto-Bismol®	Procter & Gamble
Percocet®	Endo Labs
Percodan®	Endo Labs
Perdiem®	Novartis Consumer
Peri-Colace®	Roberts
Permax®	Athena
Persantine®	Boehringer Ingelheim
Phenaphen®	Robins
Phillips Milk of Magnesia®.	Bayer
Phospholine®	Wyeth-Ayerst
Pilocar®	Ciba Vision
Plaquenil®	Sanofi Winthrop
Plendil®	Astra Merck
Polymox®	Apothecon
Ponstel®	Parke-Davis

Brand Name	Manufacturer
Posture®	Whitehall
Precose®	Bayer
Prelone®	Muro
Premarin®	Wyeth-Ayerst
Premphase®	Wyeth-Ayerst
Prempro®	Wyeth-Ayerst
Prevacid®	TAP
Prilosec®	Astra Merck
Prinivil®	Merck
Probalan®	Lannett
▲ Pro-Banthine®	Roberts
Procan SR®	Parke-Davis
Procardia®	Pfizer
Prolixin®	Apothecon
Proloid®	Parke-Davis
Pronestyl®	Apothecon
Propine®	Allergan
Propulsid®	Janssen
ProSom®	Abbott
Proventil®	Schering
Provera®	Pharmacia & Upjohn
Prozac®	Dista
▲ Quarzan®	Roche
Questran®	Bristol-Myers Squibb
Quinaglute®	Benelex
Quinidex®	Robins
Quinora®	Key
Reglan®	Robins

276

Brand Name	Manufacturer	Brand Name	Manufacturer
Relafen®	SmithKline Beecham	Slo-bid®	Rhone-Poulenc Rorer
Remeron®	Organon	Slo-Phyllin®	Rhone-Poulenc Rorer
Resphihaler®	Medeva	Solfoton®	ECR
Restoril®	Novartis	Sominex®	SmithKline Beecham
Retrovir®	Glaxo Wellcome	▲ Sominex® Formula 2	SmithKline Beecham
Rezulin®	Parke-Davis	Sorbitrate®	Zeneca
Rheumatrex®	Lederle	Sotacor®	Astra, Bristol-Myers Squibb
Rifabutin®	Pharmacia & Upjohn	Sporanox®	Janssen
Rifadin®	Hoechst Marion Roussel	Stadol®	Bristol-Myers Squibb
Riopan®	Whitehall	Stelazine®	SmithKline Beecham Pharmaceuticals
Ritalin®	Novartis	St. Joseph®	Schering-Plough
▲ Robinul®	Robins	Sular®	Zeneca
Rocaltrol®	Roche	Surfak®	Pharmacia & Upjohn
Rolaids®	Warner-Lambert	▲ Surmontil®	Wyeth-Ayerst
Rythmol®	Knoll Laboratories	SusPhrine®	Forest
Sandimmune®	Knoll Laboratories	Symadine®	Solvay
▲ Seconal®	Lilly	Symmetrel®	Dupont
Sectral®	Wyeth-Ayerst	Synthroid®	Knoll Pharmaceutical
Seldane®	Hoechst Marion Roussel	TAO®	Pfizer
Senokot®	Purdue Frederick	Tagamet®	SmithKline Beecham
Senokot-S®	Purdue Frederick	▲ Talacen®	Sanofi Winthrop
Septra®	Glaxo Wellcome	▲ Talwin®	Sanofi
Serax®	Wyeth-Ayerst	Tambocor®	3M
Serevent®	Glaxo Wellcome	Tegretol®	Novartis
Sinemet®	DuPont	Tempo Drops®	Thompson
▲ Sinequan®	Pfizer	Tenormin®	Zeneca
Singulair®	Merck & Co.	Theobid®	Russ
▲ Sleep-Eze 3®	Whitehall		

Brand Name	Manufacturer
Theo-Dur®	Key
Theolair-SR®	3M
Thorazine®	SmithKline Beecham
Thyrolar®	Forest
Ticlid®	Roche
Tilade®	Rhone-Poulenc Rorer
Timoptic®	Merck
Titralac®	3M Personal Care
▲ Tofranil®	Novartis
Tolectin®	Ortho-McNeil
Tolinase®	Upjohn
Tonocard®	Astra Merck
Toprol XL®	Astra
Toradol®	Roche Laboratories
Tornalate®	Dura
▲ Trancot®	Truxton
Trandate®	Glaxo Wellcome
Transderm-Nitro®	Novartis
Transdermal-NTG®	Warner Chilcott
▲ Transderm Scop®	Novartis
▲ Tranxene®	Abbott
Trimox®	Apothecon
Trisilate®	Purdue Frederick
Trusopt®	Merck & Co.
Tums®	SmithKline Beecham Consumer
Tylenol®	McNeil Consumer
▲ Tylenol® PM	McNeil Consumer

Brand Name	Manufacturer
Tylenol® with Codeine	Ortho-McNeil Pharmaceutical
Ultram®	McNeil
Unifiber®	Niche
▲ Unisom®	Pfizer Consumer
Univasc®	Schwarz
▲ Valium®	Roche Products
▲ Valrelease®	Roche
Vanceril®	Schering
Vascor®	Ortho-McNeil Pharmaceutical
Vaseretic®	Merck
Vasotec®	Merck & Co.
Veetids®	Apothecon
Ventolin®	Glaxo Wellcome
Verelan®	Lederle
Versed®	Roche Laboratories
Viagra®	Pfizer
Vicodin®	Knoll Labs
Viokase®	Robins
Visken®	Sandoz
▲ Vistaril®	Pfizer
Vivactil®	Merck
Voltaren®	Novartis
Wellbutrin®	Glaxo Wellcome
Wigrane®	Organon
▲ Wygesic®	Wyeth-Ayerst
Xalatan®	Pharmacia & Upjohn
▲ Xanax®	Pharmacia & Upjohn

Brand Name	Manufacturer	Brand Name	Manufacturer
Zantac®	Glaxo Wellcome	Zyflo®	Abbott
Zebeta®	Lederle Labs	Zyloprim®	Glaxo Wellcome
Zestril®	Zeneca		
Zoloft®	Pfizer		

"▲" Indicates medications that are <u>generally not recommended</u> for use in older people. Do not stop taking these medications unless directed by your doctor. They may be required under special circumstances. Talk to your doctor to see if this medication is right for you.

Resources for Help and Information

The following list is selective and restricted largely to national organizations in the United States, many of which have local chapters. Sites chosen are generally not-for-profit and usually offer information or support rather than advocacy. Telephone numbers, e-mail addresses, and web sites are included as appropriate; however, such information changes frequently. Additional information is available through health care practitioners, local libraries, telephone listings, and the Internet.

AGING

American Association of Retired People
601 E Street NW
Washington, DC 20049
800-424-3410; 202-434-2277
http://www.aarp.org

National Association of Area Agencies on Aging
1112 16th Street NW
Washington, DC 20036
202-296-8130
e-mail: jbn4a@erols.com

National Council on Aging
409 Third Street SW
Washington, DC 20024
800-867-2755; 202-479-1200
email:library@ncoa.org
http://www.ncoa,org

National Council of Senior Citizens
1331 F Street NW
Washington, DC 20004

National Institute on Aging
Public Information Office
Building 31, Room 5C27, 31
Center Drive, MSC 2292
Bethesda, MD 20892-2292
800-222-2225; 800-222-4225 (TTY);
301-496-1752
http://www.nih.gov/nia

Older Women's League
666 11th Streeet NW, Suite 700
Washington, DC 20001

ALCOHOLISM (see also Drug Abuse)

Alcoholics Anonymous
PO Box 459, Grand Central Station
New York, NY 10163
212-870-3400
http://www.alcoholics-anonymous.org

National Council on Alcoholism & Drug Dependence
12 West 21st Street
New York, NY 10010
800-NCA-CALL; 212-206-6770
http://www.ncadd.org.

ALZHEIMER'S DISEASE & OTHER DEMENTIAS

Alzheimer's Association
919 N Michigan Ave, Suite 1000
Chicago, IL 60611-1676
800-272-3900
http://www.alz.org

Alzheimer's Disease Education & Referral Center
PO Box 8250
Silver Spring, MD 20907-8250
800-438-4380; 301-495-3311
email: adear@alzheimers.org

AMPUTATION (see also Disabilities & Rehabilitation)

National Amputation Foundation
38-40 Church Street

Malverne, NY 11565
516-887-3600

ARTHRITIS

Arthritis Foundation
1330 W Peachtree Street
Atlanta, GA 30309
800-283-7800; 404-872-7100
http://www.arthritis.org

BLINDNESS & VISION PROBLEMS

American Association of the DeafBlind
814 Thayer Avenue, Suite 302
Silver Spring, MD 20910
301-588-6545 (TTY)

American Foundation for the Blind
11 Penn Plaza, Suite 300
New York, NY 10001
800-232-5463; 212-502-7600
http://www.afb.org

Association for the Education & Rehabilitation of the Blind & Visually Impaired
206 North Washington Street
Alexandria, VA 22314
no new #
e-mail: aernet@laser.met

Glaucoma Research Foundation
490 Post Street, Suite 830
San Francisco, CA 94102
800-826-6696; 415-986-3162
http://www.glaucoma.org

National Association for Visually Handicapped
22 West 21st Street, 6th Floor
New York, NY 10010
212-889-3141

BRAIN DISORDERS

National Institute of Neurological Disorders & Stroke
Office of Scientific & Health Reports
PO Box 5801
Bethesda, MD 20824
800-352-9424; 301-496-5751
http://www.ninds.nih.gov

CANCER

American Cancer Society
1599 Clifton Road NE
Atlanta, GA 30329-4251
800-ACS-2345; 404-320-3333
http://www.cancer.org

National Coalition for Cancer Survivorship
1010 Wayne Avenue, Suite 300
Silver Spring, MD 20910
301-650-8868
http://www.pageup.com/~partner/rev3

CARDIOVASCULAR DISORDERS

American Heart Association
7272 Greenville Avenue
Dallas, TX 75231
214 373-6300
http://www.americanheart.org

DEATH & BEREAVEMENT

Choice in Dying
475 Riverside Drive, Room 1852
New York, NY 10115
National Office:
1035 30th St. NW
Washington, DC 20007
202-338-9790

Dying Well Network
PO Box 880

Spokane, WA 99210-0880
509-926-2457
e-mail: Rob.Neils@ior.com
http://www.ior.com/~jeffw/dwnflyer.htm

National Hospice Organization
1901 N Moore Street, Suite 901
Arlington, VA 22209
800-658-8898; 703-243-5900
e-mail: drsnho@cais.com
http://www.nho.org

DIABETES

American Diabetes Association
1600 Duke Street
Alexandria, VA 22314
800-232-3472; 703-549-1500
http://www.diabetes.org

DISABILITIES & REHABILITATION

Disabled American Veterans
National Headquarters:
3725 Alexandria Park
Cold Springs, KY 41076
606-441-7300
http://www.dav.org

National Rehabilitation Information Center
8455 Colesville Road, Suite 935
Silver Spring, MD 20910
800-346-2742

ENDOCRINE DISORDERS

Thyroid Foundation of America
Ruth Sleeper Hall, Room RSL350
40 Parkman Street
Boston, MA 02114

617-726-8500
http://www.tfaweb.org/pub/tfa

GENERAL

The American Medical Association
515 North State Street
Chicago, IL 60610
312-464-5000
http://www.ama-assn.org

The Centers for Disease Control and Prevention
1600 Clifton Road NE
Atlanta, GA 30333
404-639-3311
http://www.cdc.gov

National Institutes of Health
9000 Rockville Pike
Bethesda, MD 20892
301-496-4000
http://www.nih.gov/science/campus

US Department of Health and Human Services
200 Independence Ave SW
Washington, DC 20201
202-619-0257
http://www.os.dhhs.gov/

US Food and Drug Administration
Office of Consumer Affairs Inquiry Information Line
301-827-4420
http://www.fda.gov

INCONTINENCE

National Association for Continence
PO Box 8310
Spartanburg, SC 29305
800-BLADDER; 864-579-7900
e-mail: sbrewer@globalvision.net

IRRITABLE BOWEL SYNDROME
Crohn's & Colitis Foundation of America

386 Park Avenue South
New York, NY 10016
1-800-932-2423
1-212-685-3440

KIDNEY DISORDERS

American Association of Kidney Patients
100 S Ashley Drive, Suite 280
Tampa, FL 33602
800-749-2257
e-mail: aakpnat@aol.com
http://www.cakp.org

LIVER DISORDERS

American Liver Foundation
1425 Pompton Avenue
Cedar Grove, NJ 07009
800-223-0179; 973-256-2550
http://www.liverfoundation.org

OSTEOPOROSIS

National Osteoporosis Foundation
1150 17th Street NW, Suite 500
Washington, DC 20036
202-223-2226
http://www.nof.org

PAIN RELIEF

American Chronic Pain Association
PO Box 850
Rocklin, CA 95677
916-632-0922
e-mail: acpa@ix.netcom.com

PARKINSON'S DISEASE

American Parkinson Disease Association
60 Bay Street, Suite 401
Staten Island, NY 10301

800-223-2732; 718-981-8001
http://www.apdaparkinson.com

PROSTATE DISORDERS

The Prostatitis Foundation
Information Distribution Center
2029 Ireland Grove Park
Bloomington, IL 61704
309 664-6222 not in service
e-mail: TCapstone@aol.com
hhtp://www.prostate.org

PSYCHIATRIC DISEASE

National Mental Health Association
1021 Prince Street
Alexandria, VA 22314
800-969-NMHA; 703-684-7722
http://www.nmha.org

RESPIRATORY (LUNG) DISORDERS

American Lung Association
1740 Broadway
New York, NY 10019
800-586-4872; 212-315-8700
http://www.lungusa.org

SLEEP DISORDERS

American Sleep Disorders Association
1610 14th Street NW, Suite 300
Rochester, MN 55901
507-287-6006
http://www.asda.org

WOMEN'S HEALTH

National Women's Health Network
514 10th Street NW, Suite 400
Washington, DC 20004
202-347-1140

Index

acarbose, 88, 89
Accolate®, 47, 48, 49
Accupril®, 156, 175
acebutolol, 144, 145, 170, 171, 196
acetaminophen, 11, 12, 13, 22, 24, 25, 140, 253, 254
acetazolamide, 94, 104
Achromycin®, 122, 123, 126, 127, 129, 130, 152, 194
Acuprin®, 257
Adalat®, 142, 143, 152, 180, 181, 194
Adalat® CC, 18, 142, 180
Adrenalin®, 31
Adsorbocarpine®, 97
Advil®, 13, 14
AeroBid®, 40
Agoral®, 58
Akineton®, 223
Alamag®, 120
albuterol, 31, 37
Aldactazide®, 168
Aldactone®, 165
Aldomet®, 80, 183, 184, 185, 186, 187
alendronate, 218
Aleve®, 14
Alka-Mints®, 120, 213
Alka-Seltzer®, 120, 122
Alkets®, 120
Alphagan®, 10, 99
alprazolam, 76, 152, 194, 236
Altace®, 156, 175
AlternaGEL®, 120
aluminum hydroxide, 120, 121

Alupent®, 31
amantadine, 229, 230
Amaryl®, 85
Ambien®, 237, 246
amiloride, 152, 165, 168, 194, amiloride & hydrochloroth-iazide, 168
amiodarone, 152, 194, 200
Amitone®, 120
amitriptyline, 65
amlodipine, 142, 180
amobarbital, 248
amoxapine, 65
amoxicillin, 123, 124, 127
Amoxil®, 123, 124, 127
Amphojel®, 120
Amytal®, 248
Anacin®, 12, 253
Anacin® Aspirin Free, 12
Anaprox®, 14
Anaspaz®, 203
Anhydron®, 162
anisindione, 251
Ansaid®, 14
Antabuse®, 129
antacid, 15, 19, 111, 117, 120, 121, 122, 152, 153, 194, 195
antidiarrheal preparations, 153
antidiarrheals, 195
Anturane®, 21, 87, 94, 253, 259
Aquachloral®, 253
Aristocort®, 27
Armour® Thyroid, 263
Artane®, 223
Arthritis Pain Formula®, 19

Ascriptin®, 19
Asendin®, 65, 112
aspirin, 11, 12, 17, 18, 19, 20, 21, 22, 25, 48, 54, 87, 94, 112, 116, 122, 125, 127, 140, 219, 253, 256, 257, 258, 259, 260,
Aspirin Maximum Strength, 19, 257
AsthmaHaler® Mist, 31
AsthmaNefrin®, 31
Atarax®, 241
atenolol, 84, 144, 145, 170, 171, 196
Ativan®, 236, 238
Atromid-S®, 87, 94, 253
atropine, 133, 203
Atropine®, 133, 203
Atrovent®, 37
Axid®, 113, 114, 115
Azmacort®, 40
Azulfidine®, 152, 194
Bactrim®, 87, 95
barbiturates, 24, 28, 44, 247, 253
Basaljel®, 120
Bayer®, 19, 257
Bayer® Aspirin Maximum Strength, 19, 257
Bayer® Aspirin Regular Strength, 19, 257
Bayer® Enteric-Coated aspirin, 19, 257
Bayer® Children's Aspirin, 19, 257
Bayer® Enteric-Coated, 19, 257
beclomethasone, 40
Beclovent®, 40

belladonna, 112, 203
Bellafoline®, 133
Benadryl®, 39, 223, 241
benazepril, 112, 156, 175
bendroflumethiazide, 163
Benemid®, 17, 21, 127, 259
Bentyl®, 203
benzodiazepines, 235, 236, 237, 238, 239
benzthiazide, 162
benztropine, 223
bepridil, 152, 194
Betagan®, 101
Betaloc®, 145, 171
betamethasone, 27
Betapace®, 145, 171, 196
betaxolol, 101, 103, 145, 171, 196
Betoptic®, 101, 103
Biaxin®, 123, 125, 128, 133
biperiden, 223
bisacodyl, 62, 112
bismuth subsalicylate, 123, 124, 127
bisoprolol, 145, 172, 196
bitolterol, 31
Blocadren®, 145, 171, 196
Brethaire®, 31
Brethine®, 31
Bricanyl®, 31
brimonidine, 99, 101
bromfenac, 14
Bromo-Seltzer®, 120
bromocriptine, 227, 229
Bronkaid Mist®, 31
Bronkometer®, 31

Bronkosol®, 31
Bufferin®, 19, 253
Bumex®, 162
bumetanide, 154, 162
bupropion, 77
Buspar®, 245, 246
Buspirone, 245
butabarbital, 248
Butazolidin®, 13, 16, 18, 87, 94, 253, 256
Butisol®, 248
butorphanol, 22
Cafergot®, 128
Calan®, 142, 143, 152, 180, 181, 194, 217, 229
Calan® SR, 142, 180, 181, 229
Calcet® Plus, 213
calcifediol, 216
Calciparine®, 255
calcitonin-salmon, 220
calcitriol, 216
calcium carbonate & simethicone, 120
calcium citrate, 213
calcium glubionate, 213
calcium gluconate, 213
calcium lactate, 213
Calcium Lactate®, 213
Calcium Rich Rolaids®, 213
Calderol®, 216
Caltrate®, 213
Cantil®, 203
Capoten®, 156, 157, 175
Capozide®, 170
captopril, 156, 157, 170, 175

Carafate®, 112, 118, 119, 122, 152, 194
carbachol, 97, 113, 116
carbamazepine, 24, 26, 36, 115, 128, 143, 182, 253
carbidopa, 225
Cardene®, 142, 180
Cardene® SR, 18, 142
Cardioquin®, 200, 229
Cardizem® CD, 142, 180, 229
carteolol, 101, 145, 171, 196
Cartrol®, 145, 171, 196
castor oil, 62
Catapres®, 183, 184, 186, 187
Celestone®, 27
cellulose, 53
Centrax®, 236
chloral hydrate, 243, 253
chlordiazepoxide, 235, 236, 238
chlorothiazide, 162
chlorpropamide, 85, 87
chlorthalidone, 163
Chlortrimeton®, 39
cholecalciferol, 216
cholestyramine, 87, 92, 153, 195, 217, 253, 265
choline magnesium, 19
choline magnesium salicylates, 19
Chooz®, 120
Chronulac®, 61
cimetidine, 36, 71, 73, 91, 112, 113, 114, 130, 133, 143, 147, 173, 182, 197, 229, 238, 253
Cipro®, 36, 119
cisapride, 113, 128, 130
Citracal®, 213

Citrocarbonate®, 120
Citrucel®, 53
clarithromycin, 123, 125, 128, 133
clidinium, 203
Climara®, 207
Climara® transdermal patch, 207
Clinoril®, 14
clofibrate, 87, 94, 253
clonazepam, 236, 238
clonidine, 67, 183
clorazepate, 236, 238
codeine, 22, 113, 115, 119, 122, 231
codeine & APAP, 22, 113, 119
Cogentin®, 223
Colace®, 55
Colestid®, 152, 194, 253, 265,
colestipol, 152, 194, 253, 265,
combinations, 33, 55, 56, 119, 122, 162, 168
Combivent®, 37
conjugated estrogen, 207, 208
Cordarone®, 152, 194, 200
Corgard®, 145, 171, 196
Cortef®, 27, 40
cortisone, 27, 40
Cortone®, 40
Coumadin®, 13, 17, 24, 48, 71, 87, 115, 117, 127, 128, 129, 130, 133, 209, 212, 244, 251, 254, 256, 265,
Creon 10®, 89
cromolyn sodium, 45
cyclosporine, 115, 128, 133, 143, 152, 182, 194
cyclothiazide, 162

Cystospaz®, 203
Cytomel®, 263
Cytotec®, 118, 119
Dalmane®, 235, 236
Daranide®, 104
Darvocet N®, 22
Darvon®, 24
Darvon® Compound-65, 24
Daypro®, 14
Decadron®, 27, 40
Decadron® Phosphate, 40
Delta-Cortef®, 27, 40
Deltasone®, 27, 40
Demadex®, 154, 162
demecarium, 97
Demerol®, 24, 25, 80
Depakene®, 20, 238, 258
Depakote®, 20, 258
Deponit®, 138
desipramine, 65
Desyrel®, 65
dexamethasone, 27, 40
DHT®, 216
Di-Gel® chewable tablet, 120,
Di-Gel® liquid, 120
DiaBeta®, 85
Diabinese®, 87
Dialose®, 55
Dialose® Plus, 55
Diamox®, 94, 104
diazepam, 71, 115, 117, 235, 236, 238
Dicarbosil®, 120
dichlorphenamide, 104
diclofenac, 15

Dicumarol®, 251
dicyclomine, 203
Didronel®, 218
diflunisal, 19, 106
digoxin, 28, 44, 89, 117, 119, 122, 128, 133, 143, 150, 151, 152, 153, 155, 164, 182, 192, 194, 195, 217, 265
dihydrotachysterol, 216
Dilacor® XR, 142, 180
Dilantin®, 17, 24, 28, 36, 44, 86, 94, 115, 117, 119, 129, 152, 194, 209, 226, 253
Dilatrate-SR®, 138
Dilaudid®, 22
diltiazem, 94, 142, 143, 180, 181, 182, 229
diphenhydramine, 223, 241
dipivefrin, 99
Disalcid®, 19
disopyramide, 200
Dispos-a-Med®, 31
Diucardin®, 162
Diurese®, 162
diuretics, 17, 21, 28, 29, 44, 86, 94, 103, 152, 153, 154, 155, 156, 158, 159, 161, 162, 163, 164, 165, 166, 167, 168, 169, 170, 175, 176, 178, 179, 194, 195, 259
Diuril®, 162
docusate, 55
Dolobid®, 19, 106
Donnatal®, 203
Doral®, 236
dorzolamide, 104

doxepin, 65
doxylamine, 241
Dulcolax®, 62
Duo-Medihaler®, 31
Duract®, 14
Dyazide®, 168
Dymelor®, 85
DynaCirc®, 142, 180
Dyrenium®, 165
E-Mycin®, 133
echothiophate, 97
Ecotrin®, 19, 257
Edecrin®, 154, 162
Effexor®, 72, 73, 74
Elavil®, 39, 65
Eldepryl®, 229, 230, 231, 232
Empirin®, 19
enalapril, 115, 116, 156, 170, 175
Enduron®, 162
enema, 57, 58
enoxaparin, 255
Epifrin®, 99
epinephrine, 31, 33, 99, 100, 101
Epsom Salts®, 59
Equanil®, 247
Equilet®, 120
Ergomar®, 128
Ery-Tab®, 36, 152, 194, 253
Eryc®, 133
erythromycin, 28, 36, 43, 133, 152, 194, 229, 253
Eskalith®, 94, 129
estazolam, 236
esterified, 207
Estrace®, 207

Estraderm®, 207
estradiol, 207
Estratab®, 207
estrogen, 114, 206, 207, 208, 209, 210, 215, 269
estropipate, 207
ethacrynic acid, 154, 162
Ethmozine®, 200
ethopropazine, 223
etidronate, 218
etodolac, 14
Euthroid®, 263
Evista®, 210, 211, 212
Ex-Lax®, 62
Excedrin®, 241, 253
Excedrin® P.M., 241
Exna®, 162
famotidine, 113, 114
Feldene®, 13, 14
felodipine, 142, 180
fenoprofen, 14
Fiberall®, 53
FiberCon®, 535
Flagyl®, 123, 125, 126, 129, 253
flecainide, 200
Fleet Phospho-Soda®, 59
Fleet's®, 57
Floropryl®, 97
Flovent®, 40, 41, 50
flunisolide, 40
fluoxetine, 70, 231, 238
flurazepam, 235, 236
flurbiprofen, 14
fluticasone, 40, 41, 50
Fosamax®, 218, 219, 220

fosinopril, 156, 175
furosemide, 91, 154, 163
Gaviscon®, 120, 152, 194
Gelusil®, 120
Genapap®, 12
Glaucon®, 99
glimepiride, 85
glipizide, 85
Glucophage®, 88, 90, 91
Glucotrol®, 85
glyburide, 85
glycopyrrolate, 203
Glynase®, 85
halazepam, 236
Halcion®, 76, 128, 236
Haldol®, 71, 186,
Halfprin®, 19
Heparin®, 254, 255, 256
heparin sodium, 254, 255
Hexadrol®, 27, 40
Humorsol®, 97
hydrochlorothiazide, 111, 116, 121, 122, 162, 168, 170
hydrochlorothiazide & capto-pril, 170
hydrochlorothiazide & enalapril, 170
hydrochlorothiazide & pra-zosin, 170
hydrochlorothiazide & propra-nolol, 170
hydrocodone & APAP, 22
hydrocortisone, 27, 40
Hydrocortone®, 40
HydroDIURIL®, 162
hydroflumethiazide, 162

hydromorphone, 22
Hydromox®, 163
hydroxychloroquine, 152, 194, 256
hydroxyzine, 241
Hygroton®, 163
hyoscyamine, 203
Hytakerol®, 216
ibuprofen, 13, 14, 112
imipramine, 65
Imodium®, 152, 194, 195
indapamide, 163
Inderal®, 36, 84, 115, 144, 145, 171, 196, 238
Inderal LA®, 196
Inderide®, 170
Indocin®, 16, 18
indomethacin, 14, 16, 18
Intal®, 45, 46
ipratropium bromide, 37, 111
Ismelin®, 94
isoetharine, 31, 116
isoetharine mesylate, 31
isoflurophate, 97
Isonate®, 138
isoproterenol, 31, 33
Isoptin®, 142, 152, 180, 181, 194, 229
Isoptin® SR, 142, 180, 181, 229
Isopto® Carbachol, 97
Isopto® Carpine, 97
Isorbide®, 138
Isordil®, 138
isosorbide dinitrate, 138
isradipine, 142, 180
isuprel, 31

itraconazole, 115, 119, 134, 152, 194
kaolin & pectin, 153, 195
Kaopectate®, 153, 195
Kemadrin®, 223
Kerlone®, 145, 171, 196
ketoconazole, 28, 36, 43, 115, 134, 238, 253
ketoprofen, 15
ketorolac, 15
Klonopin®, 236, 238
Kondremul® Plain, 58
Konsyl®, 53
Kudrox®, 120
L-Dopa, 225
labetalol, 145, 171, 172, 196
Lanoxicaps®, 119, 150, 151, 152, 192, 193, 194, 195, 217, 265
Lanoxin®, 28, 44, 84, 89, 117, 119, 122, 128, 133, 143, 150, 151, 152, 153, 164, 182, 192, 193, 194, 195, 265
lansoprazole, 116
Lasix®, 84, 91, 154, 163
latanoprost, 106, 108
Lente®, 93
Levato®, 145, 171, 184, 196
levobunolol, 101
levodopa, 78, 80, 133, 186, 223, 224, 225,
Levothroid®, 84, 263, 264
levothyroxine, 263
Levsin®, 203
Librax®, 236
Libritabs®, 235, 236, 238
Librium®, 235, 236, 238

liothyronine, 263
liotrix, 263
lisinopril, 156, 175
Lithobid®, 129
Lithonate®, 71
Lithotabs®, 71, 129
Lodine®, 14
Lopressor®, 84 144, 145, 170, 171, 196, 238
lorazepam, 236, 238
Lortab®, 22
Losopan®, 120
Losopan Plus®, 120
Lotensin®, 156, 175
Lovenox®, 255
Lozol®, 163
Ludiomil®, 65
Luminal®, 36, 129, 248
M S Contin®, 22
Maalox®, 120, 121, 130, 153, 195
magaldrate, 120
magaldrate & simethicone, 120
Magan®, 84, 19
Magnalox®, 84, 120
magnesium citrate, 59
magnesium oxide, 59
magnesium salicylate, 19
magnesium salt, 120
magnesium salts & sime-thicone, 120
magnesium hydroxide sulfate, 120, 121
Mallamint®, 84, 120
malt soup extract, 53
Maltsupex®, 53, 84
maprotiline, 65

Marblen®, 120
Maxair®, 31
Maxzide®, 168
meclofenamate, 14
Meclomen®, 14
Medihaler-Iso®, 31
Medrol®, 27, 40
medroxyprogesterone, 207, 208
mefenamic acid, 15
Mellaril®, 67
Menest®, 207
mepenzolate, 203
meperidine, 22, 24, 25, 80
meprobamate, 247
Meprospan®, 247
Metamucil®, 53, 153, 195
Metaprel®, 31
metaprolol, 172
metaproterenol, 31
metformin, 88, 90
methazolamide, 104
methyclothiazide, 162
methylcellulose, 53
methyldopa, 80, 183, 184
methylphenidate, 68, 80
methylprednisolone, 27, 40
Meticorten®, 40
metipranolol, 101
metoclopramide, 113, 130, 226, 229
metolazone, 163
metoprolol, 84, 144, 145, 170, 171, 196, 238
metronidazole, 123, 125, 129, 253
mexiletine, 200

Mexitil®, 200
Miacalcin®, 94, 220
Micronase®, 85
Midamor®, 152, 165, 194
Milk of Magnesia®, 10, 59, 120
Miltown®, 247
mineral oil, 56, 57, 58, 59, 217
Minizide®, 170
Miradon®, 251
Mirapex®, 227, 229
mirtazapine, 65
misoprostol, 118
Mitrolan®, 53
Mobidin®, 19
Moduretic®, 168
moexipril, 156, 175
Monopril®, 156, 175
montelukast, 47, 48
moricizine, 200
morphine, 22, 24, 94, 231
Motrin®, 13, 14
Mylanta®, 120, 121, 130, 153, 195
nabumetone, 15
nadolol, 145, 171, 196
Nalfon®, 14
Naprosyn®, 14
naproxen, 14
Nardil®, 24, 26, 33, 78, 79, 87, 95, 133, 226, 246
Nature's Remedy®, 628
Naturetin®, 163
nedocromil sodium, 45
Nembutal®, 248
Neo-Calglucon®, 213
Neo-Tabs®, 153, 195

Neoloid®, 62
neomycin, 153, 195
Neptazane®, 104
nicardipine, 142, 180
nifedipine, 91, 115, 142, 143, 152, 180, 181, 194
nisoldipine, 142, 180
nisoldipine, 142, 180
Nitro-Bid®, 138
Nitrocap T.D.®, 138
Nitrodisc®, 138
Nitrogard®, 138
Nitrolingual®, 138
nitroglycerin, 138
Nitro-Dur®, 138, 256
Nitroglyn®, 138
Nitrol®, 138
Nitrolin®, 138
Nitrong®, 138
Nitrospan®, 138
Nitrostat®, 138
nizatidine, 113, 114
Nizoral®, 28, 36, 43, 115, 134, 238, 253
Noctec®, 243, 244
Normodyne®, 145, 171, 196
Norpace®, 200
Norpramin®, 65
nortriptyline, 65
Norvasc®, 142, 180
NPH, 93
Nytol® Max. Strength, 241
Nytol® with DPH, 241
Ocupress®, 101
Ogen®, 28, 94. 207

omeprazole, 112, 116, 128
OptiPranolol®, 101,
oral hypoglycemics, 28, 85, 86, 87, 88, 91, 253
Orasone®, 27, 40
Orinase®, 85, 186
Ortho-Est®, 207
Orudis®, 15
Oruvail®, 15
Os-Cal®, 213, 216
oxaprozin, 149
oxazepam, 236
oxprenolol, 144, 145, 170, 172, 196
oxycodone & APAP, 22
oxycodone & ASA, 22
P.V. Carpine®, 97
Pamelor®, 65
Panadol®, 11, 12
Panex®, 12
Parlodel®, 227, 229
Parnate®, 24, 26, 33, 78, 79, 87, 95, 133, 226, 246,
Parsidol®, 223
Paxipam®, 236
PCE®, 28, 36, 43, 152, 194, 253,
penbutolol, 119, 145, 171, 196
pentazocine, 22, 24
pentazocine & APAP, 22
pentazocine & ASA, 22
pentobarbital, 248
Pepcid®, 113, 114, 115
Pepto-Bismol®, 123, 124, 125, 127, 153, 195
Percocet®, 22
Percodan®, 22

Perdiem® Fiber, 53
pergolide, 227
Peri-Colace®, 55
Permax®, 227
Persantine®, 256
Phenaphen® with Codeine, 22
phenelzine, 24, 78, 79, 87, 95
phenobarbital, 36, 129, 147, 153, 173, 195, 198, 248
phenylbutazone, 13, 14, 16, 18, 87, 94, 253, 256,
phenytoin, 17, 24, 28, 36, 44, 86, 94, 115, 117, 119, 129, 152, 194, 209, 226, 253
Phillips' Milk of Magnesia®, 59, 120
Phospholine Iodide®, 97
Pilocar®, 97
pilocarpine, 96, 97, 100, 101
pindolol, 144, 145, 170, 172, 196
pirbuterol, 31
piroxicam, 13, 14
Plaquenil®, 152, 194, 256
Plendil®, 142, 180
polycarbophil, 53
Polymox®, 123, 124, 127
polythiazide, 163
Ponstel®, 15
Posture®, 213
pramipexole, 227, 229
prazepam, 236
Precose®, 88, 89
prednisolone, 27, 40
prednisone, 27, 40, 41, 86
Prelone®, 40
Premarin®, 28, 36, 43, 94, 207, 208
Premphase®, 207

Prempro®, 207
Prevacid®, 116
Prilosec®, 112, 116, 117, 128
Prinivil®, 156, 175
Pro-Banthine®, 133
Probalan®, 127
procainamide, 115, 200
Procan® SR, 200
Procardia®, 91, 115, 142, 143, 152, 180, 181, 194
Procardia® XL, 142, 180, 181
procyclidine, 120, 223
Prolixin®, 67
Proloid®, 263
Pronestyl®, 200
propafenone, 152, 194
propantheline, 203
Propine®, 99
propoxyphene, 22, 24
propoxyphene & APAP, 22
propoxyphene & ASA, 22
propranolol, 84, 115, 116, 144, 145, 170, 171, 196
Propulsid®, 113, 128, 130, 131, 133, 134
ProSom®, 236
protriptyline, 65
Proventil®, 31
Provera®, 208, 209
Prozac®, 70, 231, 238
psyllium, 53, 153, 195
P.V. Carpine®, 97
Quarzan®, 133
quazepam, 236
Questran®, 87, 92, 153, 195, 217, 253

Quinaglute®, 115, 197, 200, 229, 253
Quinaglute® Dura-Tabs, 197, 200, 229
quinapril, 156, 175
quinethazone, 163
Quinidex®, 152, 194, 229
quinidine, 115, 147, 152, 173, 194, 197, 200, 229, 253
Quinora®, 147, 152, 173, 194
raloxifene, 210
ramipril, 156, 175
ranitidine, 113, 114, 133, 229
Reglan®, 113, 130, 131, 132, 133, 226, 229
Relafen®, 15
Remeron®, 65
Renese®, 163
reserpine, 152, 194
Respihaler®, 40
Restoril®, 236, 237
Retrovir®, 13, 128
Rezulin®, 88, 91, 92
Rheumatrex®, 20, 258
Rifabutin®, 209
Rifadin®, 28, 36, 44, 87, 147, 153, 173, 195, 198, 253
rifampin, 28, 36, 44, 87, 147, 153, 173, 195, 198, 209, 253
Riopan®, 120
Riopan Plus®, 120
Ritalin®, 68, 69, 80
Robinul®, 121
Rocaltrol®, 216
Rolaids®, 113, 120, 213
Rythmol®, 152, 194
sagrada, cascara, 121

salmeterol, 31, 34, 50
salsalate, 19
Sandimmune®, 115, 128, 133, 143, 152, 182, 194
scopolamine, 203
secobarbital, 248
Seconal®, 248
Sectral®, 144, 145, 170, 171, 196
Seldane®, 76, 92, 128
selegiline, 229, 230
senna, 62
Senokot®, 62
Senokot-S®, 55
Septra®, 87, 95
Serax®, 236
Serevent®, 31, 34, 50
Simaal®, 120
sIndocin®, 14
Sinemet®, 78, 80, 133, 186, 204, 223, 224, 225, 226, 227, 229,
Sinemet® CR, 225
Sinequan®, 39, 65
Singulair®, 47, 48
Sleep-Eze 3®, 241
Slo-bid®, 128
Slo-Phyllin®, 35
sodium bicarbonate, 112, 120, 122
sodium phosphate, 59
Solfoton®, 147, 153, 173, 195, 198
Sominex® Formula 2, 24
Sorbitrate®, 138
Sotacor®, 145
sotalol, 145, 171, 196
spironolactone, 165, 168
spironolactone & hydrochlorothiazide, 168

Sporanox®, 115, 119, 134, 152, 194
St. Joseph's® Children's Preparation, 12
St. Josephs® Adult Aspirin, 257
Stadol®, 22
Stelazine®, 39, 67, 94
sucralfate, 112, 118, 122, 152, 194
Sular®, 142, 180
sulfasalazine, 152, 194
sulfinpyrazone, 21, 87, 94, 253, 259,
sulindac, 14
Surfak®, 55
Surmontil®, 65
Sus-Phrine®, 31
Symadine®, 229, 230, 231, 232
Symmetrel®, 229, 230, 231, 232
Synthroid®, 253, 263, 264
Tagamet®, 36, 71, 73, 91, 112, 113, 114, 115, 130, 133, 143, 147, 173, 182, 197, 229, 238, 253
Talacen®, 121
Talwin®, 24
Talwin® Compound, 121
Tambocor®, 200
TAO®, 36, 134
Tegretol®, 24, 26, 36, 115, 128, 143, 182, 253
temazepam, 236, 237
Tempo Drops®, 120
Tenormin®, 84, 144, 145, 170, 171, 196
terbutaline, 31
tetracycline, 95, 122, 123, 126, 127, 129, 130, 152, 194

Theo-Dur®, 35, 115, 119, 128, 143, 182,
Theobid®, 35
Theolair-SR®, 35
theophylline, 34, 35, 36, 37, 49, 115, 119, 128, 143, 182
Thorazine®, 39, 67, 94
thyroglobulin, 263
thyroid medications, 86, 94, 253, 263, 264, 265
thyroid USP, 263
Thyrolar®, 263
Ticlid®, 256
Tilade®, 45, 46
timolol, 101, 145, 171, 196
Timoptic®, 101
Timoptic-XE®, 101
Titralac®, 120
Titralac® Plus Antacid, 120
tocainide, 200
Tofranil®, 65
tolazamide, 85
tolbutamide, 85, 186
Tolectin®, 15
Tolinase®, 85
tolmetin, 15
Tonocard®, 200
Toprol-XL®, 144, 170, 171, 172, 196
Toradol®, 15
Tornalate®, 31
torsemide, 154, 162
Trancot®, 247
Trandate®, 145, 172, 196
Transderm Scop®, 203
Transderm-Nitro®, 138, 256

Tranxene®, 236, 238
tranylcypromine, 24, 78, 79, 87, 95
Trasicor®, 144, 145
trazodone, 65
triamcinolone, 27, 40
triamterene, 165, 168, 231
triamterene & hydrochloroth-iazide, 168
triazolam, 76, 128, 236
tribasic calcium phosphate, 213
trichlormethiazide, 162
trihexyphenidyl, 223
Trilisate®, 19
trimipramine, 65
Trimox®, 123, 124, 127
troleandomycin, 36
Trusopt®, 104
Tums®, 120
Tylenol®, 11, 12, 22, 24, 25, 241, 253, 254
Tylenol® Extra Strength, 12
Tylenol® P.M., 241
Tylenol® Regular Strength, 12
Tylenol® with Codeine, 22
Ultram®, 25, 26
Unifiber®, 53
Unisom® Nighttime Sleep Aid, 241
Univasc®, 122, 156, 175
Valium®, 71, 115, 117, 235, 236, 238
Valrelease®, 235, 236, 238
Vanceril®, 40
Vascor®, 152, 194
Vaseretic®, 170
Vasotec®, 156, 175

Veetids®, 129
venlafaxine, 72
Ventolin®, 31
verapamil, 142, 143, 152, 180, 181, 182, 194, 217, 229
Verelan®, 142, 180, 181
Viagra®, 141
Vicodin®, 22
Viokase®, 89
Visken®, 144, 145, 170, 172, 196
Vistaril®, 241
vitamin K, 253, 254
Vivactil®, 65
Vivelle®, 207
Voltaren®, 15
warfarin, 13, 17, 24, 48, 71, 87, 115, 117, 127, 128, 129, 130, 133, 209, 212, 244, 251, 253, 254, 256, 259, 265
water pills, 17, 21, 29, 44, 94, 103, 152, 153, 161, 162, 175, 178, 194, 195, 259
Wellbutrin®, 77, 78
Wygesic®, 24
Xalatan®, 106, 107, 108
Xanax®, 152, 194, 236
zafirlukast, 47, 48
Zantac®, 113, 114, 115, 133, 229
Zaroxolyn®, 163
Zebeta®, 145, 172, 196
Zestril®, 156, 175
zileuton, 47, 48
Zoloft®, 70
Zolpidem, 237, 246
Zyflo®, 47, 48, 49
Zyloprim®, 36, 127, 176

PERSONAL MEDICATION RECORD

NAME: _____ PRIMARY DOCTOR'S NAME: _____ TELEPHONE#: _____

Non-prescription medications I am taking: _____ , _____ , _____

I am allergic to: _____

Name of Drug	When are you taking this medication?			With Food/ Liquid	List any problems you have with this drug	Date of Refill
	am	*noon*	*pm*	*bedtime*		

Please photocopy this table and fill it out so you can take it with you the next time you visit your doctor, pharmacist, nurse, or other health care practitioner.